MENIERE'S
AND ITS MANAGEMENT

MENIERE'S

AND ITS MANAGEMENT

By

TOM WILMOT, M.S., F.R.C.S., F.R.C.S.I.

Omagh, County Tyrone, Northern Ireland
Formerly, Consultant in Otolaryngology
to West Tyrone and Fermanagh
and in Neuro-otology to Clarement Street Hospital, Belfast
and Altnagelvin Hospital, Londonderry

With a Foreword by

David H. Craig, F.R.C.S.(Ed.), F.R.C.S.(I.)

Formerly, Consultant Otolaryngologist
to the City Hospital, Belfast
and Instigator and Founder-Member
of the Irish Otolaryngological Society

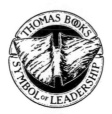

CHARLES   C   THOMAS   •   PUBLISHER
Springfield • Illinois • U.S.A.

Published and Distributed Throughout the World by
CHARLES C THOMAS • PUBLISHER
2600 South First Street
Springfield, Illinois 62717

© *1984 by* CHARLES C THOMAS • PUBLISHER
ISBN 0-398-04965-3
Library of Congress Catalog Card Number: 83-20260

Printed in the United States of America
Q-R-3

Wilmot, Tom.
Meniere's and its management.

Bibliography: p.
Includes indexes.
1. Meniere's disease. I. Title. [DNLM: 1. Meniere's
disease. WV 258 W744m]
RF275.W54 1984   617.8'82   83-20260
ISBN 0-398-04965-3

FOREWORD

TOM Wilmot came to Omagh over thirty years ago. It may be thought that it was an unusual thing for a London graduate to settle in a small county town in the middle of Tyrone, but Tom was of country stock, a most enthusiastic sportsman, and he and his wife Pat were very happy to live in the beautiful Tyrone countryside.

When he settled there he built up from nothing at all a most efficient ear, nose, and throat unit, which soon became a very busy one. For over twenty years he was a single-handed consultant, but in spite of his heavy professional commitments, and especially in his early days they were very heavy indeed, he had installed in his unit the most sophisticated modern equipment for the examination of the function of the labyrinth, and for thirty years he worked unceasingly on the problems of Meniere's syndrome.

This monograph is the result of his lifework.

In the Irish Otolaryngological Society, we were well aware of the value of the work he was doing. He has been our president, and also the president of the Otolaryngological Section of the Royal Society of Medicine in London. An unusual distinction for a surgeon from a remote part of the north of Ireland, but Tom Wilmot is an unusual man.

I think that before long this book will come to be recognised as the classic work it is.

D.H. Craig, F.R.C.S. (Ed.), F.R.C.S. (I.)

v

PREFACE

I WOULD heartily endorse Harrison and Naftalin's statement in the preface to their splendid monograph on Meniere's disease published in 1968 that pen should not be put to paper without at least twenty years experience and study of this malady. Their book is still a living testimony to their wide knowledge of the subject.

Much, however, has been published on Meniere's since then, and it now seems opportune to summarise the subject once again and to incorporate some of the modern ideas and knowledge. This book is essentially a distillation of the work of many clinicians and investigators, flavoured in doubt, as all distillates should be, with the individual ingredients, which have proved their worth in the past thirty years.

I was privileged to know, and work with, the late James Seymour during the years 1950 to 1961. His penetrating intellect and original research work kindled my interest in Meniere's. The virgin E.N.T. territory of Counties Tyrone and Fermanagh proved an ideal setting to apply his theories, then far ahead of current thinking, but our joint programme ceased abruptly with his tragic early death. Dr. Watson was left to soldier on without Sherlock Holmes — something never envisaged by Conan Doyle. At least Watson posed no serious problem to others and was able to study and oberve closely over a thirty-year period those unfortunates suffering from deafness, tinnitus, and vertigo. Although out of step with many of his professional colleagues, his idiosyncrasies were borne with toler-. ance and good humour, and he is grateful to them.

Finally, what is an expert? I do not know anyone who fits this description in relation to Meniere's — itself one of life's most fascinating jigsaw puzzles. Some of us have one piece, some more than one, and a lucky few have a conception of the whole picture. I have tried to convey my idea of this picture.

ACKNOWLEDGMENTS

I HAVE already, in the Preface, paid tribute to the late Dr. James C. Seymour, who initiated my work on this subject.

I also wish to express my deep appreciation to Franz Dittrich, the Swiss physicist, who personally designed, installed, and tested the superb and robust rotational equipment that enabled the small Tyrone County Hospital unit to engage, over a twenty-year period, in delicate vestibular function studies, without which any assessment of Meniere's disease is of doubtful value.

This equipment was operated and maintained over this long period by my chief technician, Mr. R.H. (Harry) Allen, whose consistently high standards did much to establish and maintain the reliability and reputation of the unit. In his audiometric analytical work, he showed the same attention to detail and an ability to appreciate both the technical problems and the human factors involved. In short, his judgement was of great value to me and to my patients, and I am deeply grateful to him.

I am also indebted to Dr. Keith Bosher of the Ferene Institute, Middlesex Hospital, London, whose knowledge and understanding of inner ear physiology did much to clear my mind on this complex subject.

My thanks are also due to Mrs. Phyllis McFarland, my secretary for many years, for her careful and conscientious work and to Miss Ann McKeown of Queen's University Medical Library, whose assistance in checking the references was invaluable.

Finally, it is a pleasure to acknowledge the debt I owe to the general practitioners, consultants, and colleagues of this and other areas who entrusted so many of their cases of Meniere's to my care over the years.

CONTENTS

MENIERE'S
AND ITS MANAGEMENT

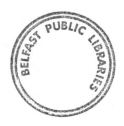

Chapter 1

INTRODUCTION

THERE is little doubt that "Meniere's disease" or "Meniere's disorder" or "Meniere's"—as it will be referred to here—poses as much a problem as it first did when described by Prosper Meniere well over 100 years ago.[169] This is remarkable in view of the enormous amount of research, both in clinical treatment and in the laboratory, that has been expended on the subject since then. Literally hundreds of articles have been published on it and related subjects, as well as a number of monographs. It has indeed now become difficult for any individual to keep abreast of all the work done and being done on this puzzling and fascinating condition.

Ingenious operations have been devised, developed, and practised on thousands of patients suffering from, or thought to be suffering from, this condition without producing any consistent results, and medical management has also failed to develop a consistently successful line of treatment. The advocates of a psychosomatic etiology have similarly failed to convince the vast majority of physicians and surgeons dealing with this condition that theirs was the correct approach.

There is further some confusion over the term *hydrops*, which many still use as being synonymous with Meniere's. While hydrops is always present to a greater or less extent in

3

Meniere's, it occurs in a number of other conditions, and it can occur without causing vertigo. Hydrops implies a pathological dilatation of part or parts of the membranous labyrinth; it does not imply a diagnosis.

The idea that the etiology of any disease can be solved by the application of modern scientific methods obtains little support from a study of the voluminous literature on this subject. Indeed, the conclusion to be reached from reading the views of many workers and authors is that two distinct possibilities exist:

Meniere's does not exist. The symptoms of deafness, tinnitus, and vertigo, which constitute the syndrome, are the result of a number of different pathological processes that disturb the function of the inner ear. Such processes may be represented by medical conditions such as diabetes, dyslipidosis, hypothyroidism, or manifestations of atherosclerosis or allergy, by mechanical factors producing failure of pneumatization of the temporal bone, by the absence, narrowing, or enlargement of the vestibular aqueduct, by stenosis of the internal auditory meatus, and by alterations of the middle ear pressure affecting the inner ear through the round window.

The proponents of this approach suggest that such findings lend plausibility to the hypothesis that Meniere's is the result of biochemical abnormalities associated with disturbed function in the inner ear.[210] Presumably correction of the etiological medical factors or surgical correction of the bony or other anatomical abnormalities should cure or alleviate the condition.

Meniere's does exist. It consists of a specific primary pathological process that is due either to an abnormality of the secretion of endolymph or to a failure in the absorption of endolymph, or to both. Amongst those who take this view there is a growing belief that psychological stress acts as the initiating, or trigger, mechanism in susceptible individuals, interfering with or disturbing normal endolymph production and *producing* the biochemical changes that are responsible for both the hydrops and the patient's distressing symptoms. They believe further that while medical conditions and minor abnormalities of temporal bone anatomy may coexist with Meniere's, they are coincidental findings and of little or no importance in the etiology. [176,177]

Complicating this picture is the fact that the symptom triad can be produced by a number of other pathological processes that involve the inner ear secondarily. These produce Meniere like syndromes and must be clearly differentiated from the primary inner ear disorder that we postulate in true Meniere's. The problem, therefore, is something akin to backache, where a few cases are due to genuine disc pathology requiring expert diagnosis and treatment but in which the vast majority are due to a multiplicity of factors that need careful assessment and evaluation. Those who believe that all backache is due to disc involvement are as incorrect as are those who believe that all patients with deafness, tinnitus, and vertigo have Meniere's. Similarly, those who deny the existence of Meniere's as an entity may be as incorrect as those who are reluctant to believe in genuine disc pathology.

The logical procedure is to review the evidence for and against Meniere's as a specific condition. This, however, is fraught with difficulties, as there is no infallible scientific test where one can designate one case as being a definite example of Meniere's and another as not filling the required criteria. Indeed, if such a test were available, this whole controversy would quickly be resolved, and there would be no need for this publication.

Even when criteria for diagnosis are considered, no general agreement obtains. Everyone has his own conception of what does and does not constitute the diagnosis. Attempts to clarify the situation by establishing both positive and negative criteria have won little support, although such clarification would appear to be both logical and essential. [283,284] In the absence of some such general agreement, it is difficult, if not impossible, to compare one series of cases with another, to assess the value of any drug treatment, or to ascertain the true value of any established or experimental surgical procedure.

  . Another difficulty lies in the psychological factors undoubtedly present in the vast majority, if not all, of these cases. The argument whether psychological problems are the result or the cause of the condition has never been completely resolved, although the weight of evidence would suggest the latter contention. Supporting this is the high, but temporary, success rate of virtually all new forms of treatment, be they medical or surgical. Even an interest shown in the patient and a thorough investigation appears favourably to react upon the patient's clinical condition.[103,104] This is yet another stumbling block in the evaluation of any treatment of Meniere's , as it results in enthusiastic acceptance of virtually all short-term follow-up regimes. Such ill-advised enthusiasm is invariably followed by a gloomy longer-term realisation that the progress of the condition has been only temporarily suspended. However, such long-term follow-up reports are conspicuously less common than their optimistic short-term counterparts and indeed are soon forgotten. In any case, other new treatments are constantly being invented and launched upon their meteoric pathways, attracting plenty of attention to them and their creators and distracting both the profession and the public from the true long-term depressing results. The idea that one of these meteors is going to be the right one is attractive, and it is both expensive in time and effort and unpopular to shoot each meteor down. It would appear, therefore, that the frequent and repeated failure of each new approach is due to a misunderstanding of the basic cause or causes of the condition.

  Much surgical endeavour is based upon the belief, which would seem to be erroneous, that there are critical anatomical and pathological abnormalities interfering with the proper absorption or drainage, or both, of endolymph and that hydrops of the labyrinth is the inevitable result. This theory implies that these abnormalities in any individual would appear to lead inevitably to the development of Meniere's and that they should be correctable surgically. If one type of operation fails to achieve long-term success, another can take its place. Repeated failure acts only as a spur to surgical invention and technique and not, except in those with genuine wisdom, to a reassessment of the underlying cause.

The assessment of results of treatment is further complicated by the extreme variability of the time interval between attacks, of the different rates of progress of the condition, of the proportion of auditory and vestibular involvement in each case, and of the incidence of bilateral disease. Because of all these factors, it is difficult even for any individual worker, analysing his own well-documented cases, to obtain more than a small series of similar cases. Each case, in fact, tends to present as an individual problem requiring individual and personal history taking and examination. Such personalized medicine is demanding in both time and experience and tends to be overlooked in many modern units where the emphasis tends to be on technical investigation and scientific assessment.

Such investigation is frequently essential in these cases, but it should be programmed to suit the individual case, and the results in each case must be assessed in light of the original history and physical findings. Emphasis should be on the quality of the technical tests and upon the quality of their assessment, rather than upon the number of cases being processed through a set programme. When the emphasis is shown to be upon strict diagnostic criteria and quality of investigation, the number of genuine cases appears to be relatively small. Conversely, series of large numbers of cases are suspect in relation to quality of investigation, diagnosis, and treatment.

In the following chapters an attempt will be made to present a picture of Meniere's that is helpful to both doctors and patients, which will discuss the various etiological theories, which will help to differentiate true Meniere's from the conditions that mimic it, and which will set out guidelines on treatment of the various stages of this perplexing and problematical disease.

Chapter 2

NATURAL HISTORY

WHILE the common and characteristic form of Meniere's is one of sudden recurrent attacks of vertigo in a patient with tinnitus and sensorineural hearing loss in one ear, the disease may present in other ways. In its very early stage (pre-Meniere's) tinnitus and a slight feeling of dizziness may be the only complaint. Sometimes the hearing loss and tinnitus may precede vertigo by months or even years, but in the majority of cases the presenting symptom is an attack of vertigo with nausea and vomiting.

GENERAL CHARACTERISTICS

Age of Onset

Meniere's occurs most commonly in the fourth decade, with three-quarters of the cases occurring between the ages of thirty and sixty.[103] Most authors agree that it is rare in small children[193,250] and uncommon in those below the age of twenty,[170,190] but Morrison states that in his experience 21 percent of his cases have commenced in childhood and that when this is the case, it is bilateral in 67 percent with all useful hearing lost in one ear in 38 percent.[181] It is also rare in the elderly, although symptoms of deafness, tinnitus, and imbalance are very common in this group due to other etiological factors.

Course of the Disease

While the common picture is of a steadily progressing disease, many variations occur. Deafness in one ear may progress slowly for years before an attack of vertigo occurs. An attack of vertigo with tinnitus and hearing loss may be followed by a long period of remission. Sometimes the attack may never be repeated. The disease may occasionally become arrested at any stage and for no apparent reason.

Total deafness, even of one ear, does not occur, although the hearing loss may be profound and the hearing in the affected ear may be of no practical significance. Bilateral deafness is also rare, although it is commoner in those who have had early bilateral involvement.[103,181]

Tinnitus is often severe and difficult to treat, especially in the later stages of the disease.

Incidence and Epidemiology

The ratio of males to females in many part of the United Kingdom appears to be roughly equal, although this varies in some areas.[103] It also varies in different countries and over relatively short periods of time.[269] In Japan, for example, it was rare before the Second World War and was more common in men (72%). Since then the disease has become much more common and is now more frequent in women (60%), in whom there is a strong likelihood of its being both bilateral and more severe (60%). The reasons for these changes are not clear, although fundamental alterations in life-style and in the emancipation of women have occurred since 1945. Also, in Japan Mizukoshi found the condition more common in white-collar workers than in fishermen and manual workers.[175]

The incidence of bilateral involvement varies in different countries but would appear to be between 10 and 30 percent in the United Kingdom.[103] Morrison, however, states that with a twenty-year history, the incidence is 45 percent.[181]

A thirty-year personal study of a relatively isolated geographical area in Northern Ireland suggests that in a community of approximately 100,000, only a small number of people will actually develop the disease, although a much bigger group will be at risk. If we consider these 100,000 people, there will be a percentage of them with a tendency to vascular instability affecting chiefly the small blood vessels. Many of these will have had chilblains when young, will suffer from migraine, from fainting attacks, perhaps from mild or definite Raynaud's disease, and even, in young women, from acrocyanosis. This percentage is probably in the region of 3 to 5 percent, that is, perhaps a total of 3,000 to 5,000 vasoactive individuals, who will also be almost exclusively hypo- or normotensive.

Out of this at-risk group will develop the vast majority of Meniere cases, who will, however, form only a small percentage of the group. The deciding factors may be linked not only with hereditary vascular tendencies but with personality as well as stress. An overconscientious, humourless individual subject to long continued, perhaps minor, stress and unable to find relief is particularly prone to become a victim.[284] Indeed, it is often "nice" people who get Meniere's, people who do not lose their tempers, who put others before themselves, who dedicate their lives to old parents, to sick children, to chronic invalids, to handicapped relatives, and so forth.

While some statistics suggest that 1 new case of Meniere's occurs annually per 1,000 population,[103] personal observation suggests that it is more in the order of 1 case per 10,000. Harrison admits, however, that much variation in the incidence rate exists. If the latter figure is realistic, then somewhere between

10 and 100 people out of our 3,000 to 5,000 at-risk group will, by bad luck, bad inheritance, inadequate personality, long continued stress, and perhaps other etiological factors develop Meniere's each year.

Although stress at work undoubtedly is responsible for some cases, domestic stress appears to be a far more common cause. The type of stress, of course, may well vary in different parts of the country and in different countries, as the reaction of different races to stress may also vary, and these variations may perhaps be in keeping with the differing incidence.

In considering our susceptible group, it is interesting that while this also contains those with allergy, vasomotor rhinitis, and asthma, who indeed form quite a large percentage of the group, it is unusual for these conditions to coincide with genuine Meniere's.

The concept of a group at risk appears to be helpful because the majority of Meniere's patients do seem eventually to fall into one of the preceding categories. The word *eventual* is used, since it is most unusual to find out the key factors in each case at the initial history taking and examination. In fact, it is only after a great deal of confidence has built up between doctor and patient that the true picture tends to emerge. A sympathetic, skilled technician, who may have to spend long periods testing an individual patient and who is infinitely less awe inspiring than a member of the medical profession, may indeed receive confidences and information that are invaluable and that might never otherwise be obtained. This is a powerful argument for allocating generous time, without external pressures, for all technical procedures.

Although the author has emphasized one type of stressful situation, obviously other varieties of stress can be important. Fowler's original suggestion of five groups is still valid.[69,70] These include personal antagonism, sexual abstinence, sexual conflicts, death of near relative, and other forms of life stress including surgical operations, tension with relatives, and financial problems.

The essential factor in all groups is the inability of the patient to cope with mounting tension — to express himself, to give way to anger, to admit that he hates someone or that he is anxious. Although they are usually of average or above-average intelligence, Meniere's cases seldom have insight into their condition until this has been made clear to them. This will be discussed later (see Chap. 7).

CLINICAL FINDINGS

In early or very early cases, tinnitus is often the first, and sometimes the only, symptom. The tinnitus may recommence or increase just before an attack of vertigo, often accompanied by a feeling of fullness on the affected side of the head or in the ear. The hearing loss too often increases before the attack.

Nausea and vomiting are characteristic of the vertigo attacks. Any movement of the head tends to exacerbate the symptoms, so the patient lies very still, afraid to move. The blood pressure is lowered, the pulse usually rapid and weak, and the skin pale and clammy. The duration of these attacks is variable, but they seldom last less than thirty minutes. Between attacks the patient may be perfectly well with no dizziness and little hearing loss or tinnitus. As the disease progresses, attacks may be more frequent, imbalance may occur between attacks, the hearing loss and tinnitus become more accentuated, and the patient becomes increasingly anxious. Migraine headaches are common in the previous history of Meniere's, and other headaches may be present in association with the attacks but are so overshadowed by the vertigo that they are seldom mentioned by the patient unless he is specifically questioned on the subject.

Vertigo

The vertigo attacks, although often sudden, are seldom sudden enough to cause the patient to fall to the ground. Usually a short warning period allows the patient to grip nearby support or to reach a chair or bed or to drive to the side of the road and stop. The attacks vary in many respects in different individuals and even in the same individual. There is often a tendency to fall laterally towards the side of the affected ear, but sometimes it is to the opposite side, and no reliability should be attached to this.

The subject of labyrinthine giddiness was described very clearly by Wright.[292,293]

Hearing Changes

In discussion of the hearing changes, Harrison states, "There is no particular type of audiometric curve which can be regarded as characteristic of Meniere's disease at any of its stages."[103] He quotes articles to support this statement with which issue must be taken.[60,191,294]

There is indeed a characteristic shape of the audiograph in *all* early cases, and this is of considerable importance in both diagnosis and prognosis. Many believe, and much evidence supports, that the first pathological cochlear changes occur in the stria vascularis and become manifest audiologically by a fluctuant sensorineural hearing loss, which always starts in the low tones. Indeed, if on the contrary the shape of the audiograph suggests a predominantly high tone loss, then even if the Meniere triad of symptoms is present it is extremely doubtful whether such a case should be included in any series of genuine Meniere's for the following reasons. First, a high tone hearing loss does not fluctuate in the characteristic way, and second, such findings are usually present in middle-aged or elderly patients with clear evidence of other pathology, often connected with cervical spine degenerative changes or evidence of atherosclerosis, which is not difficult to demonstrate.

It is perfectly true that cases of Meniere's are seen in whom the typical low tone loss is no longer present or in whom it is difficult to discern this because of spread of the cochlear lesion to involve the middle and even the higher tones. These cases are no longer at an early or reversible stage of the disease. Such findings are indeed an indication that there has been delay, sometimes a not unavoidable delay, in diagnosis. The other aspect of hearing loss that must be stressed is that while up to 20 percent of Meniere's have bilateral inner ear involvement, this *never* produces an equal or symmetrical loss of hearing.

In selecting cases of genuine Meniere's on audiological grounds, it is therefore wise to exclude all cases with a predominantly high tone loss or those with a bilateral and equal loss of hearing, whatever the shape of the audiograph. In many of these bilateral and equal high tone loss cases, the pathology is very unlikely to be due to symmetrical microcirculatory changes but is likely to be due either to advanced neural changes in the cochlea or its central connections or to macrocirculatory changes originating farther back in the arterial supply and involving both inner ears in a roughly symmetrical fashion. In this circulatory disorder cochlear damage may and does occur, and some degree of recruitment may be present, but seldom is the marked and often complete recruitment present in genuine Meniere's found in such cases.

Fullness in the Ear

Fullness in the ear, described by Alfaro in 1958,[3] occurs in about 50 percent of cases.[223] It is often accompanied by a feeling of pressure on the same side of the head and tends to be worse before an attack or during periods of frequent attacks. It is thought by some to be related to an actual increase in endolymph pressure, although it is doubtful whether this ever exceeds 1 or 2 cm of water.[26] Occasionally it precedes the onset of the other symptoms, sometimes by months or even by years[223] It is not usually present in other causes of deafness, tinnitus and vertigo, and is therefore of some diagnostic significance.

Nystagmus

Nystagmus, by which is meant clinically observed gaze nystagmus, is characteristically present in Meniere's during an attack of vertigo and for a variable period after the attack and is frequently not detectable on clinical examination between attacks. With electro-oculographic recording (electronystagmography, or E.N.G.), however, and with the eyes open in the dark, it is often possible to detect a spontaneous nystagmus between attacks. This nystagmus is brought out by the testing conditions and is best termed *latent spontaneous nystagmus*. It is usually of small degree and can be overcome by very minor stimuli acting in the opposite direction. This can be demonstrated very easily using rotational apparatus with minor acceleratory stimuli of perhaps 1° sec^2 or less. This small degree latent spontaneous nystagmus is in marked contrast to that found in cases of vestibular neuronitis.[282] In the latter condition marked gaze nystagmus is present in the early stages but disappears after perhaps ten or fourteen days, sometimes less. At this stage a powerful latent spontaneous nystagmus can be demonstrated by E.N.G. with eyes open in the dark. This requires a 3° sec^2 acceleration or even stronger stimulus in the opposite direction to overcome it.

In Meniere's whether the nystagmus is observed clinically or detected using E.N.G. as latent spontaneous nystagmus, it is usually horizontal, with or without a rotary element, and is clearly of peripheral labyrinthine origin.

While Jongkees found evidence of positional nystagmus in up to 50 percent of one series of patients,[126] Wilmot does not support this.[284] In a small series of early cases carefully selected and satisfying his positive and negative criteria for diagnosis,[283,284] he had no case with positional nystagmus. Perhaps the latter depends upon the degree of hydrops present and is only found in the well-established or late stages of the disease.

It is perhaps worth remembering that nystagmus in Meniere's, even in an acute attack, can vary greatly in type, direction, rate, and amplitude even when associated with similar pathological lesions.[19,88]

Headaches

Headaches are frequently not the almost constant or severe feature of acute attacks of Meniere's that are often depicted,[103] but the relationship between migraine and Meniere's is an interesting and frequent one. Morrison states that 30 percent of Meniere patients have migraine.[181] Many would put this figure higher than this if the past history is taken into account. A time interval, of months or even years, frequently intervenes with migraine preceding the Meniere's in the majority of those cases in which both conditions occur. This relationship will be considered further in Chapter 6.

The author has already mentioned that a sense of heaviness or fullness in the affected ear or a sense of pressure on the same side of the head, but not a true headache, is very common, and this, like the other symptoms, tends to fluctuate. It is often worse before an attack but can occur between attacks.

Psychosomatic Aspects

Many of the nervous symptoms commonly present in these cases are secondary to the distressing character of the condition. Irritability, insomnia, depression, and the like come into this category. In contrast, there is increasing evidence accumulating over many years that Meniere's is a stress-induced disease.

When we consider stress, it is important to dispel two common misconceptions. First is that it takes a very high degree of stress to produce inner ear involvement, and second is that attacks occur during the periods of heavy stress. Both these concepts are erroneous. Experience shows that a long-continued relatively minor degree of stress is associated with the development of Meniere's in many patients, and after a quiescent phase of the condition, an attack usually comes on after a further period of stress is over. When the immediate stress is over, the patient relaxes, thankful that he has had no further attack during the stressful period, only to be caught with his defences down. This happens with other psychosomatic conditions and is particularly well described in relation to alopecia.[111]

While peptic ulcertion is a common enough disorder with recognised psychosomatic etiological factors, it is interesting that this and Meniere's very seldom coexist. It would appear that if the mechanism of both is associated with the main parasympathetic nervous pathways, the harmful impulses are distributed either to the splanchnic area or to the head and neck, but not to both.

Chapter 3

PHYSIOLOGY

W HILE hydrops is not, as has already been stated, synonymous with Meniere's, it is a constant finding, to a lesser or greater degree, in the disease, and it would appear rational to focus physiological research upon the endolymph. This unique fluid provides a very real and difficult challenge to those research workers who have attempted to unravel its mysteries. The study of its secretion, electrical properties, chemical composition, circulation, and absorption require special techniques of microanalysis and micromanipulation and a vast amount of time and patience. Much of this work has of necessity to be done on animals, although human endolymph removed at operation has also been studied, and it would appear that its composition and properties are not greatly different from animal endolymph.

The results of physiological research on the cochlear and vestibular endolymph systems will be briefly outlined in the following sections.

COCHLEAR PHYSIOLOGY

It has been known for many years that the cochlea has a high endocochlear positive potential (88 mV) and that cochlear endolymph is high in potassium and low in sodium. Most of the experimental work on this subject has been performed in rats and guinea pigs, in whom the findings are almost identical. It seems reasonable to expect the human findings to be similar.

In rats the sodium ion concentration of the cochlea is 0.8 mM, the potassium ion concentration is 150 mM, and the calcium ion concentration is 30 μM (0.03 mM) in contrast to the perilymph figures of 132 mM for sodium, 6.8 mM for potassium, and 0.66 mM for calcium. This includes free protein-bound calcium, as well as very small amounts of the biologically important ionic calcium. It appears, therefore, that the cells of the stria vascularis actively pump potassium and ionic calcium *into* the endolymph and actively pump sodium (and chloride) *out* of the endolymph. Indeed, the strial cells would appear to be the only ones in the cochlea that are structurally and physiologically capable of doing this. The endolymph in the scala media with its unique composition, is not, however, static, as there is a steady leakage from this compartment, chiefly by way of the cells of the basilar membrane into the scala tympani but also to a small extent through Reissner's membrane into the scala vestibuli. It seems likely that there is a fluid and electrolyte movement throughout the boundaries of the scala media and that it is not exclusively an outward leakage but an intricate arrangement by which the ionic concentrations are maintained at the correct physiological levels. This system is not a true radial flow of endolymph as envisaged by Harrison and Naftalin, who postulated a relatively simple transference of water and electrolytes from the perilymph to the endolymph[103] but a complex system of fluid and electrolyte circulation involving the stria vascularis and the surrounding circumferential cells of the scala media.

The leakage involves the electrolytes, and since it is compensated by the action of the active transport mechanisms, it will obviously be in the opposite direction to the active transport, i.e., both into and out of the endolymph depending upon the particular ion concerned. The potassium leakage is outwards and occurs chiefly into the scala tympani. Little exact knowledge of the movements of the other ions exists.[33]

These ionic movements are primary, and if they result in osmotic imbalance, one would expect water to move in such a direction as to restore osmotic equilibrium. We do know that some or all of the endolymphatic boundaries are normally freely permeable to water.[32,257] This means that any tendency for the hydraulic pressure of the endolymph to rise or fall (as the result of any osmotic movement) will produce a hydraulic flow of water in the reverse direction to the osmotic one rather than a change in the hydraulic pressure itself. Amongst other consequences, this will make it most difficult to establish an adequate head of pressure to force cochlear endolymph along the narrow ductus reuniens (as required by the classical longitudinal flow theory).

Effect of anoxia

In the cat we know that anoxia causes a fall in the arterial oxygen level and a consequent fall also in the strial oxygen level.[171-174] This causes a reduction of the endocochlear potential, which is accompanied by a rise in the endolymphatic sodium and a fall in the potassium due to the direct effect of the anoxia on the active transport processes concerned. These endolymph composition changes produce secondary membrane changes that if the anoxia persists for ten minutes or more, greatly accelerate the rate of the electrolyte alterations.[31]

While these processes are going on, the endolymphatic calcium actually rises, probably because anoxia also causes a fall in pH, which may result in the release of bonded calcium from the tectorial membrane.[34] The rise in endolymphatic calcium results in turn in excessive calcium entering the hair cells, the vital processes of which are extremely vulnerable to this with resultant rapid derangement of their function. Relatively minor degrees of anoxia can result in impaired hair-cell activity within a short period of time, and this would provide a rational basis for the sudden onset of deafness and tinnitus in an attack of Meniere's and for the complex microcirculatory vascular supply of the cochlea, which seems ideally constructed to minimise or prevent such anoxic episodes.

Lawrence and his co-workers, in discussing oxygen reserve and autoregulation in the cochlea, point out that the blood supply to the brain and the inner ear have much in common.[146,147,149] Both systems show the characteristic of autoregulation by which is meant the ability of a peripheral vascular bed to maintain a constant blood flow over a limited range of arterial perfusion pressures.[196] This is very similar to Seymour's concept of differential sparing of the blood supply to the stria.[234]

Lawrence also showed that in guinea pigs after shutting off respiratory air the last areas in the inner ear to show oxygen depletion are the endolymph of the scala media, followed later by the perilymph of the scala vestibuli.[149] This again supports Seymour[234] and refutes the arguments of Harrison and Naftalin.[103] Lawrence concludes, "It would appear that the oxygen which diffuses into the perilymph of the scala vestibuli plays no active part in the normal metabolic or transduction processes of the cochlea."

VESTIBULAR PHYSIOLOGY

Vestibular endolymph in the utricle and semicircular canals is virtually identical to cochlear endolymph, with one important exception — it has no positive electrical potential, its potential is indeed approximately zero. In the saccule, however, the composition of the endolymph is actually determined by and depends upon the basal turn of the cochlea,[230] and this appears to result from a movement of ions along the ductus reuniens—potassium in one direction and sodium in the other—largely by diffusion with corresponding leaks across the saccular walls.

It does *not* appear to be the result of a longitudinal flow of endolymph from cochlea to saccule for two reasons.[32] First, the saccule appears to possess no cells that look as if they might be involved with electrolyte transport, and it is most unlikely, therefore, that the saccule will be able to create an osmotic gradient strong enough to pull the fluid along. Even if it could, water would move across the saccule walls rather than along the ductus reuniens. In short, there appears to be no motive force within the saccule strong enough to overcome the hydraulic pressure in the cochlea. Second, the saccule is electrically isolated from the cochlea (+ 88 mV in the cochlea against 0 mV in the saccule), and this is in keeping with the estimated resistance of the ductus reuniens of 181 k ohm. Such electrical isolation could not be maintained if there was any significent longitudinal flow from cochlea to saccule.

In contrast to the situation in the saccule, the endolymph in the utricle and semicircular canals is maintained at a constant composition by similar mechanisms to those in the cochlea, the cells concerned with the active transport being the appropriately specialised ones around the macula in the utricle and around the cristae in the canals.[231]

If for the reasons stated anoxia is a potent cause of electrolyte changes in the cochlea with resultant hearing loss and tinnitus, it seems reasonable to postulate a sudden disturbance of vestibular function (i.e. vertigo) from a similar cause.

The actual composition of endolymph in the endolymphatic sac has been difficult to estimate, but it appears to differ markedly from vestibular endolymph, having a much higher sodium concentration and a much lower potassium concentration. Estimations of endolymphatic sac endolymph have shown the sodium level to be 153 mM and the potassium level 8 mM in one study and the potassium to be 17 mM in another. These figures show radical electrolyte differences between the endolymph at either end of the endolymphatic duct and provide further strong evidence against any meaningful longitudinal flow within the system.

It seems fairly certain that the local regulation of the electrolyte composition of the endolymph in the sac is by one of the two main groups of cells present, which present the familiar characteristics indicating that they are concerned with electrolyte transport. The other main group of cells appear to be reticuloendothelial in nature and may well perform the chief function of the sac by acting as the waste bin or cleansing element of the endolymph. Whether the proteinaceous and colloid material that they remove arrives in the sac by diffusion alone or whether this is augmented by a trickle of endolymph along the endolymphatic duct has not yet been determined.

The argument that failure of endolymphatic duct drainage is responsible for Meniere's is not strengthened by experiments in animals in which the endolymphatic sac has been obliterated. While secondary hydrops has been reported many weeks or months later and minor hair-cell damage especially at the cochlear apex may occur, the weight of evidence suggests that the composition of the endolymph remains basically unchanged. Certainly electrolyte changes in the cochlear endolymph after endolymphatic duct blockage were insignificant two weeks and three months later in the paper by Morgenstern and Miyamoto.[179] Some of the late results of this type of animal experimentation may in fact be due to concomitant blockage of the venous drainage.[134,137]

In conclusion, the whole weight of physiological evidence is against the classical longitudinal flow of endolymph theory, interruption of which has been held responsible for Meniere's disease, nor is there physiological evidence to support the radial flow theory, which suggests that endolymph is formed from perilymph. There is instead evidence of a complex circulation of fluids and electrolytes both in the cochlea and the vestibule, which are vulnerable to local anoxia. It would appear logical to believe that Meniere's is due to recurrent disturbances of the regulatory mechanism controlling this microcirculation in both parts of the inner ear.

Chapter 4

PATHOLOGY

THE limitations of routine light microscopy of the inner ear are such that few contributions to the basic cause of Meniere's have come from this source since the classical papers of Hallpike and Cairns appeared describing endolymphatic hydrops.[97-99]

Some correlation between the degree and extent of cochlear dilatation and the symptomatology has been shown,[72] and cochlear hydrops without vestibular involvement has been found in cases with typical auditory symptoms without any vertigo,[40,159] but precise correlation between the degree and extent of dilatation of the vestibular system and the disturbances of vestibular function has not so far proved possible.[138] This dilatation may affect the saccule, the utricle, and both the ampullated and nonampullated ends of the semicircular canals. Perhaps as Naftalin and Harrison suggest anatomical correlation is not possible, and the vertiginous attacks result from labyrinthine fluid biochemical changes.[103] Schuknecht supported this view.[224]

In the cochlea Seymour demonstrated atrophy of the stria vascularis on the affected side in cases of Meniere's and showed that the degree of atrophy could be very pronounced even in a young patient with a relatively short history.[234] He compared this with the mild degree of strial atrophy occurring naturally in the elderly to emphasize the importance of his observations. This atrophy, most marked in the apical two-thirds of the cochlea, and its striking resemblance to the changes in severe presbycusis was confirmed by Antoli-Candela.[11]

When hydrops is severe, circumscribed outpouchings of the cochlear duct and of the membranous labyrinth occur. It would appear that these are potentially weak areas and that antemortem rupture of these herniations is not uncommon.[228] These ruptures may be associated with the attacks of vertigo; they may also lead sometimes to a perilymph-endolymph fistula. Antoli-Candela reported two cases of definite antemortem collapse of the membranous walls of the cochlear duct in two out of twenty cases. He also found suspected ruptures between the endolymphatic and perilymphatic spaces in the utricle and gaps in the membranous wall of the semicircular canals, which were sealed by a unicellular replacement membrane. The latter were usually in the posterior canal ampullae, and he felt that there was much more likelihood that they were genuine antemortem effects than the suspected ruptured areas.[11]

The hair cells are usually remarkably normal in Meniere's, even in long-standing cases with severe hearing loss.[11,224] Antoli-Candela points out that this observation is a histological one and does not imply that the cells are functional. The ganglion cells are also largely normal, although there may be changes associated with ageing,[11] and there is a direct correlation between the degree of hydrops and the level of hearing loss.

Postmortem study of the human endolymphatic duct and sac in Meniere's showed extensive fibrosis replacing the normal loose vascular tissue surrounding the sac, with varying degrees of narrowing or obliteration of the lumen, frequent collections of colloidal or proteinaceous material in the lumen, and variable changes in the epithelium.[13,222,296] These pathological changes are variable and often patchy.

The exact significance of recent electron-microscopic findings in various parts of the membranous labyrinth and endolymphatic sac is not clear.

Hydrops may also occur in serous labyrinthitis, in syphilitic labyrinthitis,[135,136,199] in inflammatory diseases, as well as in some cases of eighth nerve tumour and in conjunction with otosclerosis.[138] Syphilitic infection can cause narrowing or obliteration of the lumen of the endolymphatic duct due to granulation tissue and gummatous infiltration with secondary gross hydrops.[164]

Apical endolymphatic hydrops has been found postmortem in many temporal bones. It occurred in nearly 16 percent of 495 temporal bones where the diagnosis of presbycusis, otosclerosis, otitis media, and normal cochlea were made in approximately equal proportions.[295] It would appear, therefore, that apical hydrops is often of no pathological or functional significance. Clearly, hydrops is not specific to Meniere's, although the most widespread and severe hydrops occurs most commonly in this disease.

Gussen has also pointed out that quite marked hydrops can occur from anatomical abnormalities without causing vertigo.[96]

Electron microscopic studies in animals leave little doubt that the stria vascularis is active in fluid transport.[103] In human vestibular material removed at operation on cases of Meniere's as early as 1960, it was possible to show that the cilia of the ampullary crest are absent and that abnormal inclusion bodies are present in nerve tissue and sensory cells. The structure of the lining wall of the membranous canal suggests that here, too, there is a fluid transport system. Exfoliation of the epithelium here may interfere with the normal responses of the crista. These findings suggest that it is in the production and absorption of labyrinthine fluids that the basic cause of Meniere's lies.[198]

The chemical differences between perilymph and endolymph are well documented. Perilymph is almost certainly produced as a plasma transudate from the vessels in the lining of the bony labyrinth, either by direct passage from the capillaries of the spiral ligament or from the thin-walled capillaries of the endosteum. It is very similar to cerebrospinal fluid, except that it contains more protein than the latter. Endolymph, containing high potassium and low sodium concentrations, is probably produced by the stria vascularis, at least the cochlear endolymph is produced by the stria,[234] although the endolymph filling the semicircular canals, utricle, and saccus may be formed within these structures.[33,234]

Pollard and his co-workers state that current evidence indicates that the stria is responsible for establishing the differences in the electrolytic composition between the endolymph and perilymph[201] and quote Bosher and Warren[33] and Fernandez and Hinojosa.[62] The individual cells of the stria must actively engage in ionic transport in order to maintain the high potassium concentration in endolymph.

SUMMARY

The pathological basis of Meniere's is still far from clear. While there is limited knowledge of certain pathological changes found in this disease, there is no exact knowledge of their causation. Hydrops itself is not pathognomic of Meniere's, and its presence and degree may not be easy to correlate with the clinical findings.

Chapter 5

ETIOLOGY

A S the exact etiology of Meniere's is unknown, it seems appropriate to examine various hypotheses and see how these fit in with modern knowledge of the physiology, pathology, and clinical findings in the condition first described by Prosper Meniere.[169] As Craik in his book *Nature of Explanation* pointed out in 1943, "The importance of a theory lies not in the degree of finality attained by definition and analysis but in the power and grasp of general principles appearing in diverse instances."[49] A scientific theory should find confirmation in meeting new facts successfully, and this chapter will deal with this principle.

SEYMOUR'S HYPOTHESIS (1960)

Paroxysmal autonomic imbalance, probably initiated by a psychosomatic disorder, results in spasm of the internal auditory artery and/or its branches of distribution. The resultant diminution of blood supply causes an impairment of function of the sensory epithelium of the vestibular portion of the labyrinth if the vestibular branches are involved. This gives rise to the symptom of vertigo. The vertigo results in a fall in blood pressure through vegetative reflexes, which further increases the vascular insufficiency. Insufficiency of the cochlear vessels results in anoxia of the ganglion cells, reduced blood flow in the stria vascularis, and reduced production of endolymph, which is also qualitatively abnormal. There follows an accumulation of metabolites and a consequent increase of the osmotic pressure within the scala media, resulting in the osmotic transference of fluid from the perilymphatic and vascular compartments. The result is deafness (and tinnitus). Provided the spasm is not too severe or prolonged, recovery occurs — sometimes complete recovery — and the hearing returns to normal levels. However, if the spasm is severe or prolonged or there is frequent repetition of the attack, varying degrees of permanent damage result.

This explanation is, Seymour admits, an oversimplification of the concatenation of events that must take place. Obviously, spasm must affect other vessels too, especially those of the brain stem, and effects upon the vestibular and cochlear nuclei are also likely. These effects may influence considerably the symptoms arising from the peripheral (labyrinthine) disturbance.

Emile Meniere, the son of Prosper Meniere, suggested over 100 years ago that autonomic stimuli acting on the internal auditory artery produced vasospasm and congestion in the blood vessels of the labyrinth,[168] and Shambaugh also supported this concept.[238] Lermoyez, too, discussed the role of spasm of the internal auditory artery in vasomotor disturbances of the internal ear.[154] Shapiro, in his article "Vertigo as a Syndrome in Vascular Disease," stated, "It can be readily understood that the causes of vertigo are legion." [240] He thought that spasms occurring in the internal auditory artery or in some of the terminal vessels supplying the vestibular centres in the brain stem were the basis of most of the so-called cases of Meniere's syndrome. He also thought that a further cause of vertigo was emotional disturbances. Fowler and Zeckel also suggested that the origin of the stimulus was a psychosomatic disorder.[69,70] This has been supported by others.[43,110,124,243,256]

Hinchcliffe found that a high percentage of Meniere cases (64%) believed that their condition was emotional in origin.[110] He quotes Wolff, who in discussing the significance of psychosomatic symptoms states, "What strikes me with all these patients is that *at first* they all resist, to a greater or lesser degree, any suggestion that their physical symptoms could be emotional in origin." [288]

Hinchcliffe performed personality tests on a group of Meniere cases and contrasted them with a group of otosclerotics. He found a much higher incidence of psychosomatic personality profiles in the former.[110] Stephens supported Hinchcliffe's findings and also found a high rate of obsessionality.[256] Morrison also supports these concepts.[181]

The real question is whether this type of personality is the primary or the secondary effect of repeated attacks of vertigo,[41,91] i.e., not psychosomatic but somatopsychic in origin. Hinchcliffe points out that there is no need for the two hypotheses to be mutually exclusive. Indeed, somatopsychic effects associated with psychosomatic disorders have been recorded by several authors.[92,221] Hinchcliffe also found strong evidence of psychosomatic conditions occurring in the families of his Meniere patients.[109]

Vernet and Kobrak felt that vasoconstrictor and vasodilator effects were involved in the production of the lesions.[142,268] Hilger felt that these ideas could be compatible with sudden massive inner ear syndromes or minute insidious lesions.[107] Williams, basing his ideas on a spastic atonia of the capillaries of the stria, believed that hydrops could occur without vestibular symptoms,[273] and Lindsay reported such a case while insisting that vestibular symptoms must be present in true Meniere's. He states, "There is however strong clinical evidence that vasomotor instability may be the basis for the attacks of vertigo in most cases of Meniere's disease."[157]

Another factor that may intensify the effect of vasomotor-induced spasm in both cochlea and vestibule is the presence of blood sludging. It has been shown that autonomic stimulation produces a tendency to intravascular agglutination.[66,68] This is especially liable to happen in very small blood vessels, where the combination of spasm and sludging could readily produce a severe local anoxia. In considering the origin of the attacks of vertigo, Seymour states only that paroxysmal autonomic imbalance affecting the vestibular branches of the internal auditory artery causes an impairment of function of the sensory epithelium of the vestibular portion of the labyrinth. He does not offer any details as to the actual mechanism involved or a satisfactory explanation of its paroxysmal nature. While ruptures of Reissner's membrane or of the utricle or saccule may occur in severe cases of hydrops, this seems a most unlikely cause of the sudden vertigo in early cases with little cochlear evidence of hydrops. While it is possible that capillary blood sludging is of importance in the vestibule as well as the cochlea by accentuating the local anoxia, we still have no convincing explanation to account for the very sudden onset of many of the attacks.

Seymour stresses that, at the onset of the disease and in the early stages, all the parts of the triad may not be present and that an exact definition of the disease is neither possible or indeed very helpful, owing to "the very nature of the diversity of form of vascular disturbance, the variety of resulting physical states and the quality of human perception." [234]

That spasm of intracranial vessels can occur is indisputable. We also know from clinical observations on the lateral semicircular canal in patients undergoing operations on this structure under local anaesthesia and subjected to a cervical sympathetic block that gross dilatation of the vessels on the surface of the canal and of the supporting trabeculae of the membranous canal occurs.[194] Golding-Wood confirmed these findings in a personal communication to Seymour, proving that vasomotor control of these vessels does exist. Although under normal circumstances intracranial vessels react more actively to CO_2 concentration, metabolites, and temperature changes than to vasomotor influences, this does not apply in pathological states.[234]

Seymour also showed experimentally in cats that vasomotor control existed in the peripheral vessels in the spiral ligament and was involved in delicate control of the blood supply to the stria vascularis. He believed that this control is concerned primarily with a differential sparing of the blood supply to the stria vascularis and discussed the mechanisms involved. He stressed that the blood flow in the stria vascularis is largely regional, particularly in the apical whirls of the cochlea, and held that this accounts for histopathological changes present in localised areas of the stria, which he found in certain cases of Meniere's. He thought the same process could account for patchy distribution of lesions in the cochlea in other vascular disorders.[233]

Having established that vasomotor control of labyrinthine vessels exists, Seymour discussed the role of the sympathetic nervous system. That cervical sympathetic block can abruptly terminate an acute attack of Meniere's has been well documented.[89,122,194,234,275] It thus appeared logical to treat acute cases by a single injection of the cervical sympathetic chain and to treat cases between attacks by repeated injections[39,113] or by cervical sympathectomy.[1,53,102,122,123,156,195,275,276,278,287] The results of cervical sympathectomy will be considered in a later chapter.

Experimental work by Seymour and Tappin showed that in cats subjected to a sympathetic stimulation upon the inner ear there was a rapid reduction of the cochlear microphonics, an indrawing, or bowing, of Reissner's membrane, and histologiical changes only on the affected side in a significant proportion of the animals.[235,236] From this basis they argue that hydrops is secondary to endolymph changes — first a reduction of endolymph secretion that is qualitatively altered, resulting in an indrawing, or concavity, of Reissner's membrane. This with the resultant osmotic changes either may return to normal or, especially after repeated attacks, may result in hydrops, which in its turn may be reversible or become permanent. Cases of bilateral involvement of different degree have been described supporting this concept.[15,28,213,234]

Originally endolymph was thought to be secreted by the saccus endolymphaticus,[30] but this was challenged by Guild, whose experimental work appeared to suggest that the saccus was purely absorptive in function,[93] while Shambaugh was convinced that endolymph was secreted mainly by the stria vascularis.[237] Seymour on the basis of a painstaking histological study of animal and human material came to the conclusion that the main sources of endolymph were separate for the two parts of the labyrinth. The phylogenetically older system of utricle, semicircular canals, and saccus was supplied from the secretory tissue in the saccus, and the pars inferior, consisting of the scala media and saccule, was supplied by secretion from the stria vascularis. Normally, the utriculoendolymphatic valve separates these two systems, although Seymour found no communication in some cases without obvious other abnormalities, suggesting that the production, circulation, and absorption of endolymph is largely separate in each compartment.[233]

Although Seymour did not offer any satisfactory explanation for the unilaterality of the condition in 80 to 90 percent of those affected (this figure varies with different series of cases and in different countries), Williams suggests that the most logical explanation for the unilaterality is that the condition is due to a central stimulus. He states, "There is evidence which indicates that there are adrenergic and cholinergic hypothalamic centres and further evidence suggests that central autonomic stimuli may be unilateral." [274] Gellhorn states that autonomic imbalance is a central affair that itself depends on peripheral tuning or alteration of reactivity, not only of the autonomic nervous system but also of the other components of the autonomic system — local interface reactions, reactions of the capillary beds, and hormonal reactions. This tuning influences the autonomic centres in the hypothalamus. [79]

There seems to be general agreement that some sort of central stimulus plays an important part in Meniere's, and it may be that the hypothalamus activates the postganglionic autonomic fibres that trigger off the vascular changes in the affected labyrinth of the predisposed or susceptible individual. If such susceptibility exists, we do not know whether it is due to heredity or to a psychosomatic disorder itself possibly hereditary in origin.

Seymour's hypothesis presents a carefully argued and apparently logical case, which in its essentials depends upon the following:

1. A twin source of endolymph — the stria supplying the cochlea and saccule and the saccus supplying the utricle and semicircular canals.

2. Vasomotor disturbances — probably of central and psychosomatic origin by interfering with the microcirculation of the cochlea and vestibule being responsible for alterations of endolymph production and composition, with resultant hydrops. This process producing tinnitus and hearing loss, temporary or permanent, in the cochlea and producing vertigo in the vestibule.

3. That in many of the cases labelled "Meniere's syndrome" or Pseudo-Meniere's, the cochlea and vestibule are affected secondarily again through a vascular mechanism but *not* a primary microcirculatory one. In the majority of these cases, from whatever primary disease process they

originate, the changes are liable to affect both inner ears synchronously if not exactly symmetrically.

If we accept Craik's view that the importance of a scientific theory "lies in the power and grasp of general principles appearing in diverse instances," Seymour's theory comes through with flying colours when applied critically to the appraisal of the very wide variety of clinical conditions giving rise to deafness, tinnitus, and vertigo.

HARRISON AND NAFTALIN'S HYPOTHESIS (1968)

In their book *Meniere's Disease* Harrison and Naftalin regard Meniere's as being due to a disturbance of control both of salt and water metabolism. In the case of water, this disturbance involves a neuroendocrine secretion, itself under hyothalamic control. The changes in concentrations of salt and water, in opposing directions, are thought to exceed the limits of tolerance of the cupulae and tectorial membrane, structures highly sensitive to the state of hydration. They consider that this provides a rapid and reversible physicochemical mechanism for the acute attacks of early Meniere's. The water and salt changes are governed by a background central nervous event, which also affects the vascular supply in the inner ear.[103]

They argue that the evidence is against a longitudinal flow of endolymph from stria vascularis to saccus endolymphaticus and believe that endolymph is produced from perilymph as a type of "radial flow."[184] Perilymph, itself mainly a plasma transudate, has a high oxygen level, and they hold that it is from this source that the organ of Corti obtains its high oxygen requirement. Certainly cochlear microphonics fail quickly with oxygen deprivation[50,51] or following experimental cervical sympathetic stimulation, which also appears to cause anoxia.[235] Their argument continues that because the stria has a very high oxygen consumption (two or three times as high as the choroid plexus or kidney tubules),[44] it would be unlikely to be a good source of oxygen supply to the organ of Corti.

They say that Seymour's hypothesis is based largely on the interpretation of anatomical observations — a view that certainly does not follow from a study of Seymour's paper,[234] in which support for his theory comes from physiological, experimental, clinical, and pathological evidence.

They also throw doubt on the mode of action of cervical sympathectomy, believing that any beneficial results are due to changes in the branches of the external carotid artery, especially those small branches supplying the endolymphatic sac with a consequent increased secretion of endolymph; alternatively that sympathectomy increases the supply of perilymph with a secondary improvement in endolymph production.

Some importance must be attached to the views of Rauch on the blood flow in the spiral ligament and stria vascularis, which are at variance to those of Seymour.[211] If Seymour's "differential sparing" of the blood flow to the stria is proved correct, much of Harrison's argument may not be valid. Seymour held that this differential sparing acted as a physiological mechanism for providing a continuous good oxygen-rich blood flow to the stria and that this ensures the production of an oxygen-rich secretion — endolymph.

Harrison's counterargument states that the normal high oxygen level in the perilymph disappears rapidly during apnoea and thinks that oxygen can diffuse across into the endolymph and presumably be consumed by the oxygen-hungry stria. Even if this does occur, it does not invalidate Seymour's view that the stria is oxygen hungry because it is an actively secreting organ that gets most, if not all, its oxygen from the internal auditory artery.

Misrahy and his co-workers showed in the guinea pig that

the oxygen tension in the scala media rose as the region of the stria was approached, which supports Seymour. He also concluded from further work that the hair cells receive most of their oxygen from the stria vascularis.[171] Harrison, however, has doubts as to the degree of technical perfection possible in these situations.

While differing from Seymour on the role of the stria vascularis in the production of endolymph and the oxygen supply to the hair cells of the organ of Corti and in the way the attacks of deafness and vertigo are initiated, Harrison and Naftalin's hypothesis has several features that are in agreement with him. They specifically state that whatever happens in the inner ear "is governed by a background central nervous event which also affects the vascular supply in the inner ear." They also do not believe that hydrops is caused primarily by a failure of absorption of endolymph. Their theory, like Seymour's, does not suggest that surgery is likely to be of benefit in preventing or controlling Meniere's unless a late and nonreversible stage has been reached.

Chapter 3 pointed out that modern research does not support the concept that endolymph is formed from perilymph, although it is clear that some interchange of fluids, at a cellular level, does take place between the two fluid systems.

WILLIAMS'S HYPOTHESIS (1965)

Williams suggests that Meniere's results from a disorder of the physiological mechanism through which histamine has been shown to act as primary controller of the microcirculation in the stria vascularis. This physiological disruption may be initiated by abnormal stimuli reaching a predisposed acoustic labyrinth from hypothalamic areas tuned to autonomic dysfunction by general reactions such as emotional perturbations, hypersensitivity, and the like.[274] This hypothesis assumes that the vascular disorder in the stria is vasodilatation, not vasoconstriction, which is caused by the synthesis of histamine far in excess of its need for local homeostatic regulation. He clearly supports many of Seymour's ideas but considers he is wrong in his interpretation of what happens in the capillaries of the stria. He thinks that the changes described by Seymour and by Ireland and Farkashidy[119] actually support the hypothesis of excessive synthesis of histamine as the cause of the disorder, the histamine causing damage that results in an abnormal secretion of endolymph by the stria.

From the work of Schayer[217-220] he assumes that vasodilatation is brought about by the accumulation of toxic amounts of histamine in a free (not tissue-fixed) form in or near the vascular endothelial cells. The histamine itself is freed by the action of an enzyme histidine decarboxylase, which is always present and whose activity is responsive to changing local environmental conditions so that normally histamine is produced at the correct level to ensure normal blood flow and normal oxygenation.

Schayer states, "Increases of histidine decarboxylase activity to levels many times normal follow a large variety of stimuli, all of which may be classified as either local irritants or systemic stresses. The degree of activation of the enzyme is proportional to the severity of the stress." It would appear from this argument that induced (free) histamine produced in quantities far beyond local normal needs could produce the entire microscopic picture described in Meniere's. It would also appear that the giving of vasodilator drugs in Meniere's is strongly contraindicated—something that many clinicians would be loathe to accept. If Williams's theory is correct, it is also difficult to understand why a successful cervical sympathetic block, which must result in further vasodilatation, should improve hearing and tinnitus often within a matter of minutes and is also capable of terminating quite dramatically an acute attack of vertigo.

Williams indeed has very little to say about the origin of the attacks of vertigo. Presumably free histamine is capable of damaging the vestibular mechanism in the same way that he claims it produces the cochlear symptoms.

GUILD'S HYPOTHESIS (1927)

Guild's hypothesis is based on the belief that endolymph flows from the stria vascularis to the endolymphatic sac and that obstruction of this flow causes hydrops. He states, "If endolymph flows from the cochlear duct, as the evidence indicates, then there must be a source in the walls of this part of the membranous labyrinth. The stria vascularis is well adapted structurally for this purpose and I believe it will be found to be the principal source of endolymph in this part at least."[93] This, the "longitudinal flow theory" was supported by Lawrence[150,151] and requires either an absorptive ability on the part of the endolymphatic sac[160] or actual drainage of endolymph through the sac into the extradural tissues. The belief in an interference with this drainage mechanism being responsible for hydrops has led to the present spate of endolymphatic sac drainage operations. This was pioneered by Portman in 1927[202] and developed by House.[114-116]

The actual evidence for either absorption or drainage is scanty. In cats and monkeys the sac has no essential absorptive function,[158,229] and the experiments on guinea pigs by Guild[93] and on rabbits, cats, and monkeys by Altmann and Waltner were inconclusive.[6,7] Without conclusive proof of a true absorptive or drainage function of the endolymphatic sac, surgical attempts to provide such drainage are empirical and scientifically questionable. It is indeed doubtful whether the operation is technically feasible or ever achieves true drainage for more than a few hours or days.[227]

Guild clearly agrees with Seymour that one of the sources of endolymph is the stria. Whether there is or is not a flow of endolymph draining out of the endolymphatic sac, however, it is difficult to picture obstruction to this flow as being responsible for the attacks, often very sudden and fleeting, of deafness, tinnitus, and vertigo. Fick, however, advanced a theory that the primary cause of Meniere's was a faulty utriculoendolymphatic valve causing a buildup of endolymph with distension of the saccule and cochlear duct and that the feeling of fullness in the ear, as well as the deafness and attacks of vertigo, could be explained on mechanistic grounds. His operation of sacculotomy was based on this premise.[65] Both premise and operation have now fallen into disrepute.

Others hold that increased endolymphatic pressure and resulting hydrops cause ruptures of the system and that these ruptures coincide with the attacks of vertigo[55,148,226] by causing acute potassium intoxication and blocking of the sensory and neural elements of the auditory and vestibular systems. Such ruptures occur most commonly at the helicotrema and near the ampullae of the semicircular canals. Experimental support for this supposition was supplied by Schuknecht and Seifi in their work on cats.[229] However, such a purely mechanistic theory is difficult to correlate with the many and varied clinical patterns commonly seen.

Harrison and Naftalin review the evidence for and against the longitudinal flow theory in relation to endolymph.[103] They believe that the main source of endolymph is from perilymph and not from within the endolymphatic system itself. If this is the case, they argue that it is likely that the stria vascularis is concerned largely with absorption of endolymph, not secretion, and that the absorptive function of the endolymphatic duct and sac is relatively minor. There is, however, considerable evidence on histological and physiological grounds that the strial epithelium is secretory in nature.[88,233,234]

Further evidence against the longitudinal flow theory comes from Sadé, who describes clinical cases of extensive cholesteatomatous destruction of the area containing the endolymphatic duct and sac, in which there was no evidence of hydrops or of Meniere's disease.[216] This subject has also been considered in Chapter 3, where we have seen that the evidence is strongly against any longitudinal flow of endolymph.

OTHER HYPOTHESES

Gussen believes that the inner ear fluid mechanisms are dependent upon proper venous drainage of the vestibular organs. Increased venous pressure can in this way cause hydrops. Venous insufficiency can be brought about in several different ways to produce Meniere's, the crucial venous drainage channel being the vein of the paravestibular canaliculus (or vein of the vestibular aqueduct). This vein may be absent, predisposing to venous pressure changes in the inner ear, or it may be affected by fibrosis in the intermediate portion of the endolymphatic sac. This fibrosis is caused by fibrous tissue replacing the loose vascular tissue in the wall of the sac and is a not uncommon finding in Meniere's. The cause of the fibrosis is not known, but its effect will depend on the development of a collateral circulation. She found evidence of such in both temporal bones from a patient with Meniere's.[96]

Although she states that there has been no evidence to support the theory of a specialised cochlear microcirculation being involved in endolymph drainage, completely ignoring Seymour's work, she believes the endolymphatic sac has such a microcirculation. The properties claimed by Seymour for the cochlea she transfers to the sac, i.e., "special vessels, when stimulated by the autonomic nervous system, or specific hormones, or by as yet unrecognised factors, rapidly regulate the amount of blood contained within the organ." She believes that the melanocytes present along the vessel walls in the intermediate endolymphatic sac may be one of the regulating mechanisms of the microcirculation. If the latter is disturbed by any of the factors mentioned, a secondary rise in venous pressure occurs, and this in turn interferes with the inner ear fluid transport mechanisms.[95] The presence of malformations of the distal end of the vestibular aqueduct described in some patients with Meniere's lends support, in her view, to the critical nature of this area.[46,188,255]

Clearly, this theory is advanced as a mechanism by which different etiological processes can produce Meniere's. Although she states, "The venous insufficiency of the vestibular organs may represent the common pathway in all these conditions," we are, however, little nearer the true etiology of the disease.

Dolowitz studied the symptoms, signs, and findings in 125 cases of Meniere's. A statistical picture was then built up, and a graphic multifactor analysis suggested that the disease was of a specific central origin, or possibly several closely related diseases arising from adjacent central locations. He considered it quite likely that Meniere's is a type of inner ear seizure and felt that the unilateral ear involvement and episodic nature of the attacks supported this.[56]

There is no doubt that most of those with knowledge of the subject are agreed that a central factor is present, whether this is a stress-induced psychosomatic stimulus,[234] an ictal storm in the hypothalamus,[274] or an inner ear seizure.[56] The effective action of drugs such as cinnarazine (Stugeron®) and prochlorperazine (Stemetil®), which interrupt central impulses to the labyrinths, could be explained on this basis.

Tumarkin, in an article entitled "Thoughts in the Treatment of Labyrinthopathy," suggested that middle ear pressure changes, particularly negative pressure, might be transmitted through the round window to the inner ear to cause Meniere attacks. He advocated the use of a ventilating grommet through the tympanic membrane as appropriate treatment.[266] His argument was, however, largely theoretical, and he produced no evidence of negative middle ear pressure in Meniere cases.

Although Cinnamond studied the acoustic findings in a group of patients with Meniere's and found normal middle ear pressures and normal eustachian tube function in all of them,[45] Harker and McCabe found a higher incidence of negative middle ear pressure in Meniere subjects than normals.[101]

Tjernstrom performed experiments on human volunteers and showed that *increase* of middle ear pessure to a level of about 60 cm H_2O caused vertigo with nystagmus.[263,264] He also showed that increasing the middle ear pressure, relative to the ambient pressure, in cases of Meniere's reduced the vertigo, and he thought that this might be due either to decongestion of the inner ear or to a sudden increase in inner ear pressure causing passive forcing of a temporarily obstructed endolymphatic valve, facilitated by the decongestion. He made no comment on the relief of tinnitus or any change in hearing.

Although cases are occasionally seen in which vertiginous attacks are clearly associated with eustachian tube dysfunction, such dysfunction is clearly not present in the vast majority of patients with Meniere's, and the use of a grommet is not justifiable except as a placebo procedure.

Dolhman, who supports the longitudinal flow of endolymph theory[55] and believes that sac obstruction or obliteration can cause hydrops, in his article on the mechanism of the Meniere attack, thinks that an increase in colloid and osmotic pressure caused by cellular debris within the endolymphatic sac leads to an increased water-binding capacity of protein and that this leads to hydrops.[93]

Adour and his colleagues advanced the theory that a polyganglionitis of viral (herpes simplex) origin may be responsible by causing secondary hydrops. They describe very briefly seven cases of inner ear symptoms (labelled Meniere's) that they attribute to this cause.[2]

MENIERE'S DOES NOT EXIST AS A PRIMARY DISEASE PROCESS

Mygind and Dedering state, "Meniere's disease is not a disease *sui generis* but a typical reaction of a predisposed labyrinth to an almost infinite series of exo– and endo-genic infuences, which have, however, this in common, that they express themselves through the vessels, especially the capillaries."[183] At first sight this statement would appear to support the idea that Meniere's does not exist, but taken in conjunction with Williams's theory of excessive histamine damage and Seymour's theory of the vascular origin of the condition, it is not altogether incompatible with either of them. When does a typical localised reaction become a disease? Both Williams and Seymour accept that many factors or influences may be at work in the initial triggering of the local manifestations.

Others have considered that Meniere's is caused by other disease processes. Pulec states that a specific etiology is present in 48 percent.[205] This is denied by Moffat, who covers this subject very clearly and concisely.[176,177] He and his colleagues investigated fifty patients with Meniere's, as defined by the Committee of Hearing and Equilibration of the American Academy of Ophthalmology and Otolaryngology.[4] Each patient was tested for glucose tolerance, for thyroid dysfunction, for serum cholesterol, for triglycerides, and for allergy. The incidence of abnormal metabolic states was no higher than that of a control group. No evidence of significant allergy was found. They conclude with the following statement "This lends support to the concept that Meniere's disease is a disease in its own right."

Others, however, have reported hyper- and hypoglycaemia as causing inner ear disturbance,[104,128-130,258] and Weille reported that nearly half a small group of Meniere cases had reactive hypoglycaemia.[271]

Frequent reports of hypothyroidism associated with hearing loss and vertigo have also been made over a period of many years,[24,165,204] but hyperthyroidism is a less common cause of inner ear symptoms.[197] Hyperlipidaemia has also been held responsible,[254,273] and vitamin B complex deficiency may coexist with the hyperlipidaemia.[21] Hyperlipoproteinaemia, too, may play a part as it may itself be caused by myxoedema, renal disease, diabetes, obesity, and heavy nicotine consumption.[253,254]

Moffatt and his colleagues also discuss the role of allergy acting possibly through arteriolar spasm and anoxia of the stria vascularis to produce the auditory symptoms, and similar spasm in vessels supplying the cristae and maculae to produce the vertigo, but they found no evidence of allergy in the group they studied.[176,177] Food sensitivity—both fixed and cyclic types—may be another etiological factor.[212]

Although there is no doubt that other disease states may coexist with Meniere's, there is little real evidence that any one disease or any combination of diseases has a constant role in the etiology. It may indeed be that these varied pathological processes produce inner ear symptoms of the Meniere type because secondary damage to the cochlea and/or vestibule occurs. The mechanism may be, in all or most of these conditions, a vascular one, but one which does not primarily involve the microcirculation.

The other condition that is common, which frequently results in some involvement of both cochlea and vestibule and which is very important in the differential diagnosis because it occurs frequently in the same age group as Meniere's, is degenerative arterial disease. That manifestations of atheroma may interfere with cerebral and inner ear circulation is obvious. Indeed, many middle-aged and elderly patients present with inner ear symptoms before they develop clear evidence of circulatory problems in their coronary arteries or branches of the vertebrobasilar system. Seymour was one of the first to draw attention to this, and he felt that this was not evidence of the nonexistence of genuine Meniere's but, on the contrary, strong supporting evidence of a true vascular etiology in Meniere's. He felt that such cases were basically of macrocirculatory origin, as distinct from the primary microcirculatory lesions present in true Meniere's. Vertebrobasilar insufficiency is certainly often associated with inner ear symptoms, but in this and in all the varying conditions that cause secondary deafness, tinnitus, and vertigo, a psychosomatic factor is conspicuous by its absence.

There is no doubt that Meniere's is much commoner amongst the white races. Whether this is genetic or associated with stress that is more common in developed societies is uncertain. We know that it is very rare in Negroes,[80] and this has also been reported in relation to the Bantus in South Africa[64] and in Jamaicans.[20] Indeed, the condition is so uncommon that Black considered that two cases occurring in a West Indian male and a West African female were worth reporting.[29]

It is interesting also that Meniere's has become much more common in Japan since the Second World War, and the previous predominance of males has altered to nearer the European norm.[185] These findings might be construed as additional evidence of the presence of a central psychosomatic precipitating factor associated with the industrialisation of a previously rural society and with the changing role of women in Japanese society.

SUMMARY

The weight of evidence would appear to suggest that Meniere's is a specific disease process and not just the result of a reaction of the inner ear to multiple etiological factors. If we accept this, we are faced with the problem of finding a satisfactory working hypothesis that fits into the complex pattern of cochlear and vestibular symptoms and signs that constitute this condition. It seems reasonable to start by excluding those theories which are based on purely mechanistic concepts, i.e., alterations of middle ear pressures that produce secondary inner ear effects and obstructions of endolymphatic flow by congenital or acquired abnormalities of the endolymphatic duct or sac. Clearly the evidence for either of these theories is scientifically invalid; moreover, both theories fail to answer many more questions than they do answer.

It seems unlikely also that Adour, who postulates a viral cause, has found the answer[2] or that Dohlman has added much to the obstructive endolymphatic sac hypothesis.[55]

Ruth Gussen's theory of venous drainage impairment is interesting and may well play a part both in predisposing to the condition and in affecting the degree of involvement of both cochlea and vestibule, but it, too, leaves many questions unanswered.[95]

We are left, therefore, with the theories of Seymour, Harrison and Naftalin, Williams, and Dolowitz, in all of which there is agreement that a central factor is involved. The nature of this factor is ill understood, but psychosomatic impulses acting through the hypothalamus, producing largely unilateral inner ear effects, seem to have some general support. These effects are almost certainly produced by microcirculatory changes in the cochlea and vestibule. In our brief analysis of modern physiological knowledge of endolymph production and composition, it would appear likely that minor degrees of anoxia affecting the main production areas of endolymph, i.e., the stria vascularis and the maculae of the utricle and saccule, could, by creating rapid ionic concentration changes, produce rapid alterations in both cochlear and vestibular function. Whether this occurs through a primary vasoconstriction or a primary vasodilation and whether free histamine is or is not involved appears relatively unimportant at this stage of our knowledge. What is important is that our attention be focused on the vital role played by the microcirculation in maintaining the endolymph in its normal physiological role.

The idea that there is a longitudinal or a radial flow of endolymph appears to be erroneous, and quite clearly the whole process of endolymph production and control of its constituents is complex, involving both selective pumping in of some ions and pumping out of others, as well as leakage of both water and other constituents from the scala media. While water and salt metabolism is certainly involved,[103] potassium, calcium, and magnesium are also involved in a continuous process upon which the functions of the hair cells and of the vestibule depend. Clearly, early changes are often relatively slight and reversible. Unchecked damage becomes progressive and irreversible.

In conclusion, it would appear that the general consensus is drifting toward accepting the views of Seymour and Williams that a psychosomatic or central stimulus operating in susceptible individuals through a vasomotor mechanism to create microcirculatory changes that induce endolymph abnormalities is the essential mechanism in producing Meniere's. This theory certainly provides the clinician with an explanation of the vast majority of cases of Meniere's, both in the modes of onset, the variable progression, the different degree of involvement of cochlea and vestibule, the fluctuating symptoms, the early reversibility and later irreversibility, and the response to treatment dependent upon the stage to which the disease has progressed. In short, if logically applied, it does provide a working hypothesis strong enough and pliant enough to guide both patient and medical adviser in a manner that is both hopeful and, in most cases, extremely satisfactory. In support of this, Golding-Wood lists thirteen conditions that must be met to make any hypothesis tenable. He examines each of these in relation to Seymour's hypothesis and finds clinical and/or experimental evidence in support of them all.[88]

Chapter 6

DIAGNOSIS

FICK writes, "Meniere's disease is too often diagnosed and very often misdiagnosed."[65] This has certainly been the case in the past and may well still be true. Until relatively recently, the diagnosis has been made largely on clinical grounds and often without the elimination of other more common causes of inner ear symptoms. Wilmot has repeatedly pointed out that the diagnosis should not be presumptive but should be reached by a process of elimination.[283-285] If it is assumed that symptoms of deafness, tinnitus, and vertigo are *not* due to Meniere's, one will be far more often right than wrong. If progress in understanding this condition is to advance, very rigid diagnostic criteria must be established and agreed upon, both nationally and internationally, so that proper comparisons may be made between different groups of cases. This should lead, in time, to much better assessment of the results of treatment — medical, surgical, or placebo — and ultimately to much more consistent success in treatment.

The Committee of Hearing and Equilibration of the American Academy of Ophthalmology and Otolaryngology defined Meniere's in 1972, which was a big step forward.[4] It is doubtful, however, whether their definition was rigid enough for present needs, as it is still possible for a series of patients with deafness, tinnitus, and vertigo to be labelled as Meniere's when up to 48 percent of them are shown to have these symptoms as part of another disease process.[206]

Although technical improvements, particularly in the field of audiology, have recently brought some degree of scientific confirmation of the cochlear lesion in Meniere's, vestibular testing techniques have not yet reached this degree of sophistication, although Wilmot points out that considerable progress has been and is being made in this direction.[284]

Both auditory and vestibular testing refinements have been limited, in the United Kingdom, to a small number of special units, with the result that in the nonspecialised units covering the greater part of the country the diagnosis of Meniere's is still made upon the history, clinical findings, simple pure tone and speech audiometry, and the caloric test. This may be perfectly adequate where the standard of audiometry is high and where the clinician responsible for each case is prepared to spend considerable time and trouble; however, it is certainly not adequate unless these conditions are met. Obviously, technical confirmation of both cochlear and vestibular lesions is highly desirable. In all units, however, it is important to consider in some detail how the making of the correct diagnosis may be improved.

PATIENT HISTORY

There is little difficulty in understanding the symptom of hearing loss and in communicating with the patient on the subject. Tinnitus, too, although present in some variation, is a relatively problem-free subject for discussion between patient and medical adviser, as is the sensation of fullness in the ear or side of the head, of which many patients with Meniere's complain.

It is in dealing with the subject of vertigo that real difficulty arises, due to the problem many patients have in describing their giddiness. Gowers defined vertigo as "any movement or sense of movement, either in the individual himself, or in external objects, that involves a defect, real or seeming, in the equilibrium of the body."[91] This definition is hard to fault or to improve. Clearly he saw vertigo as a wide range of symptoms containing true rotational vertigo but not confined to it.

If we accept this definition, then we must also accept that there are a large number of patients with some sensorineural hearing loss, tinnitus, and a balance disorder who do not have typical Meniere's. These patients must be differentiated from Meniere's and they must be investigated properly and treated accordingly. Meniere himself noted, as have all others with long-term experience of the disease, that one or other of the main triad of symptoms could appear many years before the others and that there were often long intervals of remission between the attacks of vertigo. Both these factors complicate the diagnosis.

In taking the patient's history, it is helpful if some system is applied; otherwise, vital information may not be elicited. While allowing the patient some freedom to tell his own story in his own words, and he may have some difficulty in doing this, it is important that the examiner have a coherent plan in his own mind to follow in each case. The following programme is suggested:

First, the clinician must obtain a detailed account of the onset, type, severity, duration, and frequency of the attacks of vertigo, and in particular the relevant details of the very first attack, if this can be recalled. He should note what the time of onset was, whether the patient was resting or in bed; and whether it came on after violent exertion, in conjunction with migraine or other severe headache, in association with influenza, after a head injury, after an ear operation, after a particular form of drug therapy, after a period of severe psychological trauma or prolonged mental, emotional, or physical stress, after travelling by air, or after diving or underwater swimming or exertion. The onset of vertigo after some of these activities, while mimicking Meniere's, may well be due to entirely different causes, so these questions may be of crucial diagnostic significance.

Is the giddiness associated with a sense of rotation, either of the surroundings or of the patient himself? Is it accompanied by nausea or vomiting? Was nystagmus noticed? Does movement of the head during the attack exacerbate the symptoms? Does the attack only come on when the head is in a certain position? Can the patient foretell an attack? Is any food thought to be responsible? The answers to these questions quickly help the examiner to build up a mental picture of the type, degree, frequency, and possible origin of the attacks.

The date of onset of the deafness should be noted, whether it is unilateral or bilateral, whether it fluctuates, whether it is progressive or is accompanied by excessive noise intolerance or distortion or by alterations of pitch perception. Does the deafness increase before or during an attack of vertigo? For example, in the Lermoyez syndrome, increasing deafness and tinnitus is followed later by a paroxysm of vertigo, after which the hearing returns.[154,155] Golding-Wood agrees with Lermoyez that this type of attack is due to vasospasm affecting the internal auditory artery and that the sudden release of spasm results in the return of hearing.[88] Both Golding-Wood and Williams consider that this is but a variant with the same pathological mechanism as Meniere's.[273]

Previous deafness from other causes may also be unilateral or bilateral and may be secondary to old or present middle ear disease. A chronic discharging ear with severe hearing loss may cause vertigo through direct involvement of the bony labyrinth.

Tinnitus in the hearing-impaired ear may be continuous or

intermittent, low or high-pitched, or of "white noise" type. It, too, may and usually does vary with an attack of vertigo. It is commonly present as a low tone intermittent tinnitus in Meniere's *before* there is appreciable subjective loss of hearing or any vertigo, i.e., it may be the first symptom. It is therefore important in the diagnosis of the early reversible stage of this condition. A high-pitched tinnitus is more suggestive of other cochlear or neural pathway pathology. A feeling of pressure or fullness in the ear or side of the head is common in genuine Meniere's and seems to be more common in those who are getting frequent attacks of vertigo. It may be directly related to the degree of hydrops present.

Next, questions should be directed towards conditions affecting the head and neck that might give useful differential diagnostic information. This is particularly important in relation to headaches, epilepsy, visual or other sensory defects, reduced neck mobility, and pain or tenderness on neck movement.

There is a close association between headaches and Meniere's. Several authors have testified to the connection between migraine and Meniere's.[21,37,88,108,109] Hinchcliffe states, "Examination of patients' histories seems to indicate that whilst in early adult life they suffered from episodes of migrainous type headaches, in middle adult life these headaches became replaced by episodes of vertigo." Many would agree with him. Migraine itself is well documented as being of psychosomatic origin.[74,131,162]

It is interesting that migraine headache is the characteristic headache in Meniere's. Other types of headache do occur but not in the same association, and they do not have the same diagnostic vaue. It is important to remember, too, that migraine may have a definite vertiginous aura with nausea and vomiting.[57] Morrison points out that although migraine has a strong positive family history, he found a positive family history in Meniere's in only 2.6 percent.[181] Mizukoshi, however, puts the figure at 5.5 percent.[175] The aura of epilepsy also may be associated with vertigo, particularly if the symptoms of brain failure come on relatively slowly.[57]

The importance of neck symptoms lies in two main conditions—"cervical vertigo"[36,52,187,215] and the role of cervical spondylosis in vertebrobasilar insufficiency. That cases of vertigo are precipitated by neck movements in some cases is not in doubt. The exact mechanism, however, is not at all clear.

The general health of the patient may be very relevant, particularly as regards a history of hypertension, angina of effort, obesity, diabetes, circulatory problems, or thyroid or renal disease, all of which may be responsible for, or contribute to, inner ear symptoms that mimic Meniere's. Paroxysmal auricular fibrillation especially is one cardiac condition that should be kept in mind, and postural hypotension is another uncommon but very genuine cause of giddiness. Personal habits in relation to nicotine and alcohol may give valuable clues also in the diagnostic process.

Whilst this history taking is in progress, the opportunity to assess the personality of the patient should not be missed. This may contribute a missing piece to the complete jigsaw puzzle that constitutes the correct diagnosis.

Stress vertigo undoubtedly occurs, both in children, where it often presents in association with examination nerves, and in adults, usually young adults. The symptoms are purely vestibular.

The overconscientious individual with unresolved and sometimes unresolvable problems is particularly prone to genuine Meniere's.[283] Finally, the patient's occupation should not be forgotten, as this sometimes plays a part in the etiology and may give both a clue as to diagnosis and help later in management.

PHYSICAL EXAMINATION

The physical examination of the patient must include the mobility of the cervical spine, the presence or absence of gaze nystagmus and of discobolos, and an examination of the cranial nerves and optic fundi. A positive discobolos test — the extended arms in the seated patient swinging to the side of the labyrinthine lesion when the eyes are closed — and a positive past-pointing test are usually found when gaze nystagmus is present, which will of course have its fast component in the opposite direction. Peripheral (labyrinthine) nystagmus is usually horizontal and unidirectional. Central nystagmus is usually multidirectional. If it is unidirectional, it beats to the side of the lesion, which is often present in the posterior fossa.

In assessing the circulatory system, the pulse and blood pressure should first be taken. The latter should be taken in both arms to exclude a subclavian steal syndrome, which can also cause inner ear symptoms.[120] If a 30 mm pressure difference is present, this condition should be excluded by angiography.

If the history is suggestive of a postural hypotension, the blood pressure should also be taken, both lying and standing. A failure of the pressure to rise when the patient stands confirms this. Next, the carotid arteries should be palpated, and cold extremities and acrocyanosis noted as well as the degree of nicotine finger staining.

Obesity can be important, as can anaemia and evidence of thyroid imbalance. Signs of heavy alcohol consumption should not be missed. The urine should be tested.

The ears and hearing must then be examined clinically, and the otologist will exclude other E.N.T. disease before deciding the type and nature of the audiometric tests required. Finally, a simple clinical assessment of the patient's balance while sitting, standing, and walking should be made. Balance tests should include the Romberg test, single-leg standing, heel-toe walking along a marked straight line, and walking with eyes open and closed. A tendency to fall to one side consistently suggests a recent peripheral vestibular lesion. Generalised unsteadiness or an atypical gait is often associated with a cerebellar lesion, but there is usually no consistent directional falling.

The defense of equilibrium test, which should be done with discretion, consists of standing behind the patient, who is gazing at a point straight ahead and suddenly tipping both his shoulders backwards towards the examiner. This can give valuable information in nonorganic vertigo when the reaction is exaggerated but effective and in central lesions when the reaction is largely absent.

Time spent on the initial history and general physical examination is nearly always time saved,[124] as it is upon these initial findings that a decision on the whole pattern of future and perhaps highly specialised investigations will depend, the results of which must or should harmonize with the simple clinical background.

After preliminary clinical assessment and after routine audiometry has been performed, and before embarking on a wide range of auditory and vestibular tests, it is sometimes wise to obtain a consultant medical, neurological, or psychological opinion.

AUDITORY EXAMINATION

Routine air and bone pure tone audiometry and speech audiometry establish both the threshold of hearing and the shape of the hearing curve. The clinical diagnosis of a sensorineural hearing loss is also confirmed. The next necessity is to establish whether recruitment is, or is not, present, and the loudness discomfort test is quick and effective.[112]

Low tone loss of hearing for pure tones in the affected ear, together with low-tone tinnitus (which can be matched on the audiometer) with definite evidence of recruitment and excellent speech discrimination, is characteristic of most, if not all, early cases of Meniere's. The picture may change as the disease progresses, but the emphasis should always be on early detection and early treatment. Significant tone decay does not occur. The findings are therefore typical of an end-organ (cochlear) lesion commencing towards the apex of the cochlea.

It is relevant to emphasize that in very early cases the hearing loss may be very minor indeed, perhaps 10 decibels in the lower frequencies, but this always coincides with the side of the tinnitus and with any evidence of recruitment if such can be demonstrated.

Appreciation of these points helps in recognising the stage of the condition at which the patient seeks advice. This is clearly very important if an early diagnosis is to be made, which is fundamental to a good prognosis. The stages that are clearly recognisable are as follows:

1. Very early   — Reversible
2. Early   ⎤
3. Intermediate   ⎦ — Partially reversible
4. Established   ⎤
5. Late   ⎦ — Nonreversible
6. Bilateral

Technical advances in objective audiometry have come from the acoustic impedance meter, from Békésy audiometry and from electric response audiometry. With impedance audiometry, recruitment can be demonstrated in the hearing impaired ear very satisfactorily by utilising the stapedial muscle reflex at known suprathreshold levels. Békésy audiometry usually shows a typical Jerger Type 2 chart in Meniere's disease, confirming a peripheral cochlear lesion.

The most useful form of electric response audiometry in the differential diagnosis of Meniere's is transtympanic electrocochleography, initiated by Portmann and his co-workers in 1967,[203] which records the electrical events occurring within the cochlea and the eighth nerve in response to various sound stimuli. It can be used to study the electrophysiological changes in different diseases. The compound eighth nerve action potential/summating potential (AP/SP) wave form has been shown to be widened in cases of Meniere's.[81] The exact reason for this is not known but may be due to displacement by hydrops of the cochlear partition with resultant asymmetry in the mechanoelectrical phenomena associated with hair-cell stimulation. The summating potential also increases during periods of increased hearing loss in the fluctuating stage of Meniere's. As fixed hearing loss develops, however, the summating potential tends to decrease, so a study of the summating potential may be of value in assessing what the degree of cochlear involvement is and whether it is reversible or not.[47,82] Characteristic changes also occur in eighth nerve tumours.

Brain stem evoked responses also produce diagnostic variations in both Meniere's and eighth nerve tumours.[232] This technique has the advantage of being noninvasive and is used in some units in conjunction with or to replace electrocochleography. Absence of brain stem responses is an early finding in a large percentage of cases of multiple sclerosis. This can be of considerable differential diagnostic value, as these absent responses are found even with virtually normal pure tone and speech audiometry, such as may occur in a very early case of Meniere's or in multiple sclerosis. Two other procedures can give valuable information about the reversibility of cochlear auditory function and of cochlear duct hydrops, and thus help in deciding the stage of the disease.

The Glycerin Test

The ingestion of glycerin by mouth described by Klockhoff and Lindblom[140] and Klockhoff,[139] which acts as an osmotic diuretic, frequently produces a temporary improvement of the hearing in the affected ear in cases of Meniere's in its early and intermediate stages but not in other conditions. Klockhoff hypothesises that glycerin produces an intracochlear hydrodynamic damping effect, either directly by decreasing the amount of endolymphatic hydrops and intralabyrinthine pressure or indirectly by lowering the perilymphatic pressure.[33] It gives a positive reaction in over 60 percent of Meniere's and is a useful confirmatory test.[249,262] Presumably the percentage of positive reactions will depend upon the percentage of relatively early cases in any series.

It has been shown recently that glycerin actually increases the cochlear blood flow, which may be the mechanism behind a positive result.[145] There is, however, no exact knowledge whether this increase in blood flow is generalised throughout the cochlea or localised to the stria vascularis. Morrison points out that it is important with this test to confirm dehydration by showing a rise in plasma osmolality of at least 10 mM/litre one to one and one-half hours following the ingestion of 1.5 ml glycerin/kg body weight. Confirmation of reduced hydrops is obtained by pre- and post-glycerin testing with the otoadmittance bridge. This shows a positive change in the maximum conductance following the glycerin, which is in keeping with the improvement shown in the pure tone and speech audiograms.[181]

Futaki and his co-workers believe that the diuretic furosemide is a better agent than glycerin and that it produces much fewer side effects.[76]

Cervical Sympathetic Block

Testing for cervical sympathetic block effects can be of

diagnostic value, as it, too, can produce shifts of auditory threshold. These shifts are characteristically upwards in cases of early and intermediate Meniere's. In cases of hypertension or atherosclerotic inner ear symptoms, on the other hand, they are often downwards. First advocated by Passe and Seymour as both a diagnostic and therapeutic procedure,[195] it has enjoyed popularity and unpopularity since then.

If satisfactory sympathetic release is obtained by the procedure and a good Horner's syndrome results, it is common for auditory pure tone thresholds to rise by 10 to 20 decibels, especially in the low tones (250, 500, and 1,000 Hz), and for tinnitus to be much diminished or banished. These effects are, of course, usually only temporary. Cervical sympathetic block during an acute attack of Meniere's can rapidly abort the attack.[89,275]

VESTIBULAR EXAMINATION

The profession has been slow to realise that the caloric test, however performed, gives inadequate information for the differential diagnosis of vertiginous lesions in the vast majority of cases.[285] There is now growing appreciation that a number of tests are required, as in auditory analysis, to obtain the requisite information about the vestibular system. Although the process of auditory analysis has now largely been standardized and is accepted internationally, the same cannot be said about vestibular analysis.[279,284] Principles, however, are being established, and it is only a question of time before a standard routine is established. This should include clinical balance tests, positional tests, neck torsion tests, optokinetic and eye-tracking tests. The semicircular canals should be tested both by bithermal (caloric) and angular acceleratory stimuli, using rotational[178,277,279,283,284] and/or torsion swing equipment,[121] and the otolith organ should be tested by the parallel swing.[189] Obviously, the use of this whole battery of tests is not necessary in every case, and it is up to the clinician to ensure that the patient is not overtested and that the team is not wasting valuable time.

It is appropriate to describe some of the common vestibular test findings:

OPTOKINETIC NYSTAGMUS. Optokinetic nystagmus is usually normal with a peripheral vestibular lesion, as in Meniere's, although there may be some directional preponderance shown with electronystagmographic (E.N.G.) recording in keeping with the side of the lesion. When central nystagmus is present, it is usually unaffected by the optokinetic stimulus.

POSITIONAL NYSTAGMUS. If strict diagnostic criteria for Meniere's are adopted and early cases are being considered, positional nystagmus is usually absent.[284] If present, it is usually of the fatigable benign type. It may be related to the stage of the lesion, as Jongkees found it present in 50 percent of one series.[126] Positional vertigo (cupulolithiasis) is well covered by Schuknecht.[225]

A persistent central positional nystagmus suggests a lesion of the vestibular nuclei.

NECK TORSION NYSTAGMUS. If neck torsion in a particular direction produces consistent nystagmus, it is suggestive of cervical vertigo. This type of nystagmus is characteristically absent in Meniere's.

EYE-TRACKING (FOLLOWING) TEST. The eye-tracking test is usually done by asking the patient to follow the swing of a pendulum with his eyes. This is normal in Meniere's. Abnormalities of eye tracking occur characteristically in lesions of the brain stem associated with neurological disorders such as Huntington's chorea, progressive supranuclear palsy, and familial ataxia, but arteriosclerosis and vascular accidents can also be responsible and may coexist with inner ear symptoms.[54] With all of these vestibular tests, it is important to realise that successful results are almost directly proportional to the amount of time and attention to detail that the technical team can spend with each individual patient. Selectivity is thus of paramount importance, and this is clearly the otologist's, or neuro-otologist's, responsibility.

The belief that electronystagmographic (ENG) recording would simplify the investigation has proved fallacious. While it has certainly enhanced the interest of the subject, it has also increased its complexity both in relation to testing methods and their interpretation. Indeed, there is still argument whether caloric tests should be done with or without E.N.G.[16] Without E.N.G., duration of the nystagmus, with optic fixation, is the only measurement possible, and the difficulty here is in deciding the end point. With E.N.G., and without optic fixation, emphasis is laid upon the speed of the slow nystagmic component or upon the eye shift per second, rather than upon the duration of the nystagmus. If a latent spontaneous nystagmus is present, which it often is using E.N.G., the duration of the nystagmus may be difficult to estimate and is not a true estimation of the caloric response.

A valid criticism of the bithermal caloric test is that it provides a single relatively powerful stimulus with each thermal test. Unless there is considerable loss of semicircular canal function a normal, or near normal, reaction ensues. With rotational or torsion swing testing a range of stimuli can be used, and the reactions plotted against these. This provides considerable diagnostic information and is of particular importance in early lesions.[284] Considerable technical skill is required in all tests done with E.N.G., and constant vigilance has to be exercised both in their performance and in the supervision of the equipment. Computerised readouts of the test material have done much to save laborious methods of measuring nystagmus, but they are by no means standard equipment and may, without careful supervision, give misleading information.

At the end of every testing programme, it remains the clinician's responsibility to analyse each patient's results, to interpret them, to integrate them with the clinical history and clinical findings, and to make a diagnosis. The final step, of course, should be to talk to the patient and make a firm decision about treatment. This all sounds fairly simple, but the more complex the testing procedures the more difficult it is to relate the results back to the individual patient. Every neuro-otological unit must pay particular attention to this aspect if it is to fulfil its proper function.

RADIOLOGICAL AND OTHER SPECIAL INVESTIGATIONS

An acoustic neurinoma may need exclusion. While the presence of recruitment and the absence of tone decay is 65 percent accurate in this exclusion,[192] tomographs improve this accuracy to 90 percent,[133] and brain stem evoked response audiometry further increases this to 95 percent.[58] Hypocycloidal polytomography is also a useful diagnostic procedure,[22] particularly before contemplating endolymphatic sac surgery, as it is held by some authors that Meniere's is linked with the following physical abnormalities.

1. The pneumatisation pattern of the temporal bone is said to be decreased.[143]
2. The position of the endolymphatic sac is said to be more caudal, more medial, and more anterior than normal, lying often medial to the descending course of the facial nerve. The sac is also said to be shorter and straighter than normal.
3. Nonvisualisation of the vestibular aqueduct is common.[255] The aqueduct is also said to be narrower than normal and

may be a hereditary disorder.[188,200]

1. Primary basilar impression may be present.[38,186] This may not only be the factor responsible for the difficulty in visualising the vestibular aqueduct within the temporal bone,[132] but it is said to be responsible for Menierelike symptoms.[59]

Finally, blood serum tests to exclude syphilitic infection are important.[135,136,199,247] When such infection involves the membranous labyrinth and cochlea, it can cause hydrops and mimic Meniere's very closely. This subject is well covered by Becker[25] and by Belal and Linthicum.[27]

DIFFERENTIAL DIAGNOSIS

The history, physical examination, and analysis of the hearing loss and of the loss of vestibular function will in most cases provide clear clues as to the correct diagnosis. The conditions that may commonly be mistaken for an acute atack of Meniere's in its different stages are as follows:

1. Vestibular neuronitis, which is recognized by the absence of any cochlear involvement and by characteristic findings on rotational testing of vestibular function.[282]
2. Migraine when accompanied by vomiting and dizziness. Visual symptoms, paraesthesia, speech disorder, or limb weakness suggest brain ischaemia from migraine. There is usually no cochlear involvement. The vertigo may be intense and rotatory and of the same quality as an attack of Meniere's.[57] It is not infrequent in children.
3. Epilepsy. Sometimes a well-marked vertiginous aura occurs, and the patient than falls, not from the vertigo but from the epileptic brain involvement.
4. Transient cerebral ischaemic attack. This, like migraine, can cause genuine rotational vertigo. Such an attack

commonly occurs in the middle aged or elderly and is associated with degenerative arterial disease.[240] Because many of these patients have also some difficulty in hearing and perhaps some tinnitus, the differentiation between this type of degenerative macrocirculatory type of inner ear involvement from genuine Meniere's presents considerable difficulty. It is this group of patients who tend to swell the numbers of reported cases of Meniere's in many series.

In these cases the hearing loss is usually most marked in the high tones and is frequently symmetrical or almost symmetrical. Recruitment is often present but to a lesser degree than in Meniere's. Tinnitus is usually higher pitched than in Meniere's. The vertigo is usually less episodic than in Meniere's, and there is often a slight residual imbalance between attacks, which is usually not present in Meniere's.

It will be seen that in considering purely the deafness, tinnitus and vertigo confusion may arise, but other clues to the true etiology are not difficult to find. Hypertension, cervical spondylosis, obesity, diabetes, evidence of heavy nicotine and/or alcohol consumption, and so forth are commonly present. Indeed, the presence of such findings should militate against a diagnosis of Meniere's.

5. Acoustic neurinoma. This is much rarer than any of the preceding conditions. It should be suspected in all unilateral cases of sensorineural deafness and systematically excluded. Tone decay tests, electric response audiometry, and special radiological techniques will confirm the diagnosis. Caloric tests are of little value in the diagnosis of early acoustic neurinomata.

6. Ramsay-Hunt syndrome. This again is rare. Vestibular symptoms and cochlear symptoms may accompany the herpes zoster rash on the auricle and the facial nerve

paralysis. The vertigo may be very acute with a persistent nystagmus initially of third degree and gradually subsiding. Caloric tests show a marked directional preponderance, which again lessens gradually over several weeks. Sometimes the vertigo is much less severe. The sensorineural hearing loss may be severe and permanent or less severe and reversible.

7. Disseminated (multiple) sclerosis. A single episode of lasting giddiness is not uncommon with genuine rotatory vertigo. Repeated lesser attacks may occur. Cochlear symptoms are much rarer. Electric response audiometry using brain stem evoked responses show characteristic changes.

8. Perilymph fistula. The symptoms and signs may closely mimic Meniere's. It not infrequently follows trauma, surgical or accidental, and follows a fluctuating course. When a patient is thought to have Meniere's but behaves in atypical fashion, a perilymph fistula should be suspected. Fraser and Flood have recently described an audiometric test that proved positive in a high percentage (five out of seven) cases. A pure tone air conduction and a speech audiogram are done. The patient then lies down with the affected ear uppermost for one-half hour. The audiographs are repeated with the patient still lying down. A 10-decibel pure tone rise in at least two frequencies or a significant gain in speech discrimination is significant.[71]

9. Metastases. Occasionally secondary deposits from malignment tumours may, by involving the inner ear directly or the region of the internal auditory meatus, produce inner ear symptoms that mimic Meniere's. In the majority of cases the clinical history will draw attention to this possibility. Secondary deposits in the brain stem are unlikely to affect hearing and balance only.

SUMMARY

Essential to the diagnosis of Meniere's is a comprehensive history and a good clinical (medical rather than surgical) examination. Auditory analysis is now a routine worldwide procedure and should confirm the typical recruiting peripheral (cochlear) lesion present. Such analysis now includes electric response audiometry. Vestibular analysis is also essential, and progress in this direction has commenced.

While special radiological techniques may show abnormalities in the bone structure in Meniere's, these should be treated with reserve until more is known about the true etiology.

A brief description of the conditions commonly simulating Meniere's is included.

Chapter 7

TREATMENT

FROM the numerous hypotheses that have been advanced and have been considered to be responsible for Meniere's, it is obvious that little or no general agreement has been reached on treatment.[125,265] The situation is further complicated by the lack of agreement on the exact criteria for diagnosis and is compounded by little appreciation, until recently, of the importance of suiting treatment to the various stages of the disorder. In short, it is difficult to find amongst all the physicians and surgeons treating Meniere's two who are likely to agree upon details of treatment. Although many will agree upon a principle of treatment, these principles are based upon the individual's concept of the etiology, so there are widely differing views on how to treat the disease in keeping with the differing etiological theories.

While some favour a salt-restricted diet, others favour drugs that suppress the symptoms, drugs that are thought to improve the microcirculation of the inner ear, or drugs that restrict histamine liberation in the stria vascularis. The control of vasomotor instability is the aim of some, while others believe that control of sugar metabolism or correction of allergy is all important. Others again consider that stress has a vital primary etiological role and that its correction must have priority.

Some again are interested in the very early and reversible stages of this condition; others do not see patients with really early symptoms. Again, some surgeons are concerned with the results of their careful, meticulous, and precise surgery, others are more concerned with their operative statistics or the financial rewards of surgery. Many ingenious operations have failed to cure the condition, although they have done much to widen our surgical horizons.[65,152,214]

The multifactorial problem that has been briefly outlined is still further compounded by the very nature of the condition itself, which is characteristically intermittent, inconsistent, and frequently unpredictable. It is against this background that the published results of treatment have to be assessed and evaluated. It is not surprising that the personal integrity of the reporting physicians and surgeons assumes considerable importance. There is perhaps general agreement that all patients should have an initial period of medical treatment and that surgery is normally reserved for those who have not responded to this. The indications for, and the timing of, operative treatment, as well as the type of operation, will be considered later.

Management of a patient complaining of tinnitus, deafness, and vertigo is dependent upon an accurate assessment, and this aspect has been emphasized under diagnosis. Perhaps the first essential in management is a good patient-doctor relationship.[94,124] The foundations for this should have been laid very soundly during the initial assessment period. All these patients, and their relatives, are worried, and they are profoundly reassured by the degree of interest shown, by the thoroughness of the history taken, and by the physical examination made. These are indeed the fundamentals upon which all subsequent management is built.

It is essential, therefore, that a high quality team be built up to handle all aspects of the diagnosis and treatment of each case. This will include nursing care and assistance, technical investigation, personal medical involvement at general practioner and consultant level, and a first-class communication system involving all those necessary for these tasks and for the continued supervision of each case.

This team will be committed to every case with inner ear symptoms, whether the final diagnosis is Meniere's or some other disorder. It will require a high degree of organisation if the results achieved are to be commensurate with the total effort involved. The person responsible for this organisation is the otologist or neuro-otologist in charge of the unit.

This approach should be concerned with the personality and the problems of the patient as much as with the actual inner ear symptoms, i.e., the holistic approach, one which is now gaining favour in many fields of medicine[105] and in the approach to Meniere's.[245,272]

Under these conditions it should be possible to make an early, or even a very early, diagnosis and to institute early efficient total management. This should largely obviate the need for surgery. Conversely, the failure of medical management, even at an early stage of the disease, may call for early surgical intervention. It is thus artificial to discuss management under the separate headings of medical and surgical, as both medical and surgical skills may be needed by the team in the actual physical management of many cases of Meniere's. It is important to understand that commonsense psychological management is essential also.

Many patients with Meniere's have difficulty both in describing their symptoms and in finding a doctor who understands and can discuss these with them. Patients often have a shrewd suspicion as to the cause of their troubles, and a history and examination that does not bring out these suspicions, correct or incorrect, is incomplete. This book has already emphasized the reassurance that a thorough history and examination can give to the patient, not only relieving anxiety but helping to transfer the load from patient to doctor. Simple reassurance after an inadequate assessment does not achieve this object in the same way, certainly not with an intelligent patient, and patients with Meniere's (like those with migraine) tend to be of average or above average intelligence.

If we accept that stress has an etiological role in the majority of, if not all, patients, it is extremely important that each patient must be given insight into the way that stress can initiate both the disease itself and individual attacks of vertigo. Specialised psychiatrists or psychotherapists are not necessary. Counseling at this stage can be done quite simply by the general practitioner, otologist, or physician responsible for the case. This is especially true in the early stages of the disease, when the condition is still reversible. Many of these patients are overconscientious[283,284] or somewhat obsessive[256] and because of their personalities and a particular life situation, they have often not had a proper holiday, at least from the long-continued stress, for years. This should be rectified as a matter of urgency.[283,284]

Ideally, it should be possible to see and diagnose each case early and to restore physiological and psychological balance before the inner ear has been irreversibly damaged, but this will depend upon a very efficient referral system, upon education of the public to seek early specialist advice, and upon education of the profession to ensure that patients with very early or early symptoms are properly investigated and treated.

If the disease has progressed to a nonreversible stage, it is still important that the patient be given insight into the way that stress can exacerbate the attacks. Support should not be on a day-to-day basis but as a long-term commitment that strategic advice will be available at intervals over a period, if necessary, of years. The day-to-day management should largely be in the hands of the patient himself with the help of his general practitioner, who should be fully brought into the picture.

Management of the different stages of Meniere's will now be considered. This should comprise psychological, physical, and supportive elements in each case and at each stage of the disease, although the emphasis will vary depending upon the stage of the disease when the diagnosis is first made.

VERY EARLY MENIERE'S
(PRE-MENIERE'S) – STAGE 1

Tinnitus, usually low toned, and a very slight unilateral hearing loss confined often to the frequencies below 1 kHz may be the only symptoms of early Meniere's. A feeling of dizziness may also have occurred but seldom a real attack of vertigo. These cases should be fully investigated without delay; they should not be reassured and sent away, allowing the disease to progress.

Psychological management is most rewarding at this stage, by removal, if possible, of the long-continued stressful situation, which is usually the precipitating factor, and is emphasized by the taking of a holiday. Nicotine addiction may have an adverse effect and should be eliminated. Mild sedation may be indicated, and a suitable vasodilator drug such as betahistine (Serc®)[286] should be given in large doses (6 to 12 mg four times daily) for at least six weeks. An alternative drug at this and later stages of the disease is thymoxamine (Opilon®) (40 to 80 mg three or four times daily),[84] and Thomsen and his co-workers advocate lithium treatment.[259]

Total reversibility and long-term cure should be the aims of treatment at this stage. Cynics might suggest that these very early symptoms and signs are unconnected with genuine Meniere's, but careful questioning reveals that many advanced cases have indeed gone through this early stage, not without complaint but frequently without much help, on their way to the fully developed syndrome. If the patient can be given real insight into the way he reacts to stess and some simple advice as to what to do if at some future period the symptoms recur, the long-term prognosis at this stage is excellent.

The question of dietary control should also be considered early in the course of the disease. Salt and water restriction was first advocated by Furstenberg[75] and still has its advocates and opponents.[87] Weille, however, points out that this soon results in renal conservation of sodium with increased loss of potassium. He suggests it is more logical to suppress aldosterone activity and to give a thiazide diuretic to ensure a renal loss of water and soidum and a consequent *retention* of potassium. The level of serum potassium must, of course, be monitored.[270] These measures should certainly be considered if early reversal of symptoms does not occur or if there is a recurrence.

EARLY MENIERE'S — STAGE 2

Early Meniere's is the earliest stage at which most cases are referred to the consultant. A definite hearing loss, always in the low tones, that fluctuates and is accompanied by a low-tone tinnitus and a feeling of fullness in the ear, also of a fluctuant nature, are the presenting symptoms. One or more attacks of real vertigo have occurred with nausea and vomiting, or the patient may have had only dizzy spells that tend to be associated with an increase in the tinnitus and hearing loss.

Between attacks of vertigo, it may be difficult to assess each clinical situation, as the hearing may be almost normal and the tinnitus absent. Management is basically the same as for the very early case but will depend upon

1. The duration of the disorder
2. The degree of fluctuation and of potential reversibility
3. The recognition of this stage of the disorder

4. The ability to neutralise the precipitating emotional or other primary etiological factor
5. The mode and effectiveness of treatment

In some cases of Meniere's still at this stage, there may be a relatively long history, but little permanent damage to cochlea or vestibule may have occurred. In these cases neutralising the precipitating factor setting off the attacks may be the most efficient way to stop further attacks. This would appear to act by correcting the presumed vasomotor instability.

If the patient is seen during an acute attack, this is the ideal time to perform a cervical sympathetic block.[88,122,194,234,287] Immediate relief of vertigo with reduction or cessation of tinnitus and improvement in hearing commonly results. This is of considerable psychological benefit to the patient, who then appreciates that his condition is reversible, and indeed, sometimes the rapid relief of symptoms is followed by a long period of remission.

A cervical sympathetic block may also be useful between attacks. Again elevation of the hearing and reduction of tinnitus often result. The hearing gain is usually of the order of 10 to 15 decibels and is confined to the frequencies of 250, 500, and 1,000 Hz. Sometimes there is a gain of 25 to 30 decibels.

The injection for cervical sympathetic block is best done by the lateral route (Fig. 1) The patient should be lying supine on a couch with the head turned slightly to the opposite side and supported by a pillow (or an assistant) in such a way that the neck is neither flexed nor extended. Imaginary tangents are drawn AB and AC (Fig. 2), and the needle is inserted where the tangents meet and vertical to the skin at this point, which in the normal or thin neck is two fingers breadth (4 cm) above the clavicle. The needle, which should be fine and short bevelled, is directed toward the transverse process of the sixth cervical vertebra. When it strikes the bone, usually at a depth of 4 to 6 cm, it should be withdrawn 4 or 5 mm, aspiration to exclude blood or cerebrospinal fluid performed, and the injection made. Two or 3 ml of 1% solution of procaine or lignocaine is injected. With the needle still *in situ*, the patient is then sat bolt upright, and the solution is allowed to gravitate. The aim of the injection is not to inject the stellate ganglion itself but to insert the fluid into the correct tissue plane (this will require very little syringe pressure), where it can run down towards the ganglion. With correct technique it is frequently possible to get an excellent Horner's syndrome with as little as 2 ml in as little as two minutes.

When the subject has a short thick or fat neck, it is wise to insert the needle higher in the neck but with the same tangential angle, sometimes as much as 2 or 3 cm higher. In these subjects the depth to the sixth transverse process may be considerable, and the aim is to get the injected fluid onto the fifth or even the fourth cervical transverse process. Gravity will do the rest. A direct approach by this route to the stellate ganglion involves the needle's traversing the apex of the lung in many cases and is inadvisable. If a Horner's syndrome does not start to develop rapidly, a further injection, up to a total of 5 ml, is made through the needle already in position.

The degree of sympathetic release is variable. It is often striking, but occasionally, in spite of an accurate technique it is disappointing and appears to be related to the individual. With good sympathetic release, a marked flush of the conjunctiva and of the vessels of the tympanic membrane of the ear on the injected side is seen. The hearing level and the degree of tinnitus should be assessed immediately before and thirty minutes after the injection. If different technicians are employed to use the same audiometer and if the levels are done blind, there is less likelihood for any bias in the results.

The injection can also be done by the anterior route,[103] and this has been commonly used. The lateral route, however, has many advantages. With the anterior route method, paralysis of

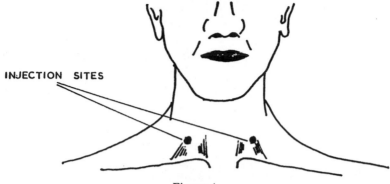

Figure 1.

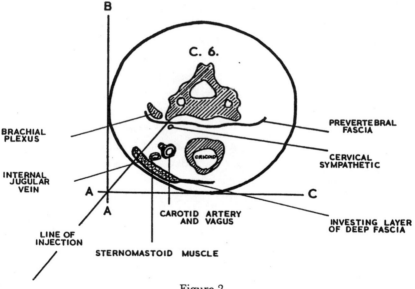

Figure 2.

the recurrent laryngeal nerve is not uncommon.

Sometimes oral glycerin[139,140] or oral furosemide[76] can be used as a therapeutic, as well as a diagnostic, measure. Larsen and his colleagues have shown that glycerol actually increases cochlear blood flow, although it is not known whether this increase is a generalised one or affects principally the stria vascularis.[144,145] The chief disadvantage of taking glycerin is the severe headache it frequently provokes, and its repeated use is contraindicated.

Gibson and his coworkers gave intravenous naftidrofuryl (Praxilene®) and found that it controlled the vertigo and reversed the characteristic electrocochleographic changes found in Meniere's.[83] Klockhoff has also given chlorthalidone (Hygroton®) orally 100 mg/day for one month in a single dose, reducing to 50 mg/day and stopping after two months freedom from vertigo. With frequent recurrences, they gave 50 mg every second day as continuation therapy. They claim that this is useful in controlling symptoms in ambulant patients and that in a series of 220 patients it avoided operation in 60 percent. The side effects are usually slight, but sometimes excessive exhaustion and fatigue are produced even with small doses, and the drug has to be stopped.[141]

Although there are some practical disadvantages to the use of diuretics as a form of treatment, cervical sympathetic block can be repeated as necessary and has been used successfully as a form of treatment.[39,113] If such treatment fails ultimately to arrest or reverse the disease, cervical sympathectomy is a logical sequel. This will, however, very rarely be necessary in the type of early Meniere's that is now being considered.

It must be emphasized that the strategy of management at this stage is directed toward discovering the degree of reversibility present and in bringing about as great a reversal as possible. Time in this stage of Meniere's is vital, and everything should be done, as quickly as possible, to ensure that the disease does not progress to an irreversible state.

Drug treatment should not be prolonged unless satisfactory progress is being made. It certainly should not replace the line of general management already outlined, although it can complement it. There is yet no wonder drug that acts specifically to counteract Meniere's, and considering the complexity of the subject, this is not surprising. Betahistine certainly has a part to play at this stage, but it must be given in adequate dosage at least three and preferably four times a day up to a total of 48 mg/day. The hearing and tinnitus should be carefully monitored at regular intervals, and the drug discontinued at the end of six to eight weeks if material improvement in symptoms and signs has not resulted.[286] Whether this drug acts by increasing strial blood flow or by limiting histamine release in the cochlea, it has been shown by several investigators to give better than placebo results in clinical trials,[73,106,280,281,286] and this is supported by studies in animals that showed vasodilatation of capillaries, arterioles, and arterial venous arcades in the stria vascularis and spiral ligament following betahistine therapy.[163]

Betahistine has few side effects,[286] although it does sometimes cause indigestion and may have to be discontinued for this reason. It should not be given to patients with a history of peptic ulceration, fortunately a very rare finding in Meniere's. Other vasodilator drugs such as nicotinic acid and thymoxamine can be used as an alternative to betahistine, but the same principles should apply.[84]

It is doubtful whether the labyrinthine sedatives such as prochlorperazine maleate (Stemetil®), cinnarizine (Stugeron®), promethazine theoclate (Avomine®), dimenhydrinate (Dramamine®), or buclizine hydrochloride (Equivert®) should be used at this stage of this disease except to control acute attacks of vertigo or for brief periods to ensure symptomatic relief. The latter must *not* be bought at the price of disease progression.

If the previous management regime has been applied conscientiously and on the basis of full assessment and accurate diagnosis, the prospect of arresting the disease is good, and there is a fair chance of reversal, or partial reversal, of the hearing loss and tinnitus and cessation of the vertigo. It should certainly ensure a long remission period in most cases. If a relapse occurs later, repeated treatment along the same lines may again produce remission, but late relapse usually implies a failure to eliminate the causative stress and is often associated with further progression of the disease.

If, however, all endeavours are in vain and it is clear that the condition is not under control and that stage 2 is becoming stage 3, the question of surgery must be considered.

INTERMEDIATE MENIERE'S — STAGE 3

Definite hearing loss, still predominantly low toned, is now present, and the hearing does not return to normal during fluctuations or as the result of treatment. Vertiginous attacks of some severity occur at frequent or infrequent intervals. Tinnitus and a feeling of fullness in the affected ear are both troublesome.

The principles of psychological and physical management are again deployed. The degree of reversibility, by cervical sympathetic block or glycerin test, is assessed, and the effects of intensive drug therapy are observed and monitored. Sometimes such patients can be stabilised at this level or even improve enough to be relabelled stage 2, but for the most part some irreversible damage is present, and progress towards stages 4 and 5 is likely. It is at this intermediate stage that a decision to operate or not to operate can be very important and very difficult. The hearing loss is usually not great, so a destructive operation is contraindicated. In addition, of the operations that conserve hearing, only vestibular neurectomy is relatively sound. Vestibular neurectomy, however, is a major operation requiring great technical skill and expertise. The alternatives are cryosurgery[117,290] and ultrasonic irradiation of the vestibule.[8-10,17,18,244,251,252] While the results of these less invasive procedures have been generally favourable, they have also been somewhat unpredictable and unreliable. Facial paralysis is not uncommon and has been reported as high as 10 percent after cryosurgery.

It is at the intermediate stage, and indeed also in Stage 4 (the fully established disease), that many surgeons have resorted to endolymphatic sac surgery.[5,12,14,35,46,114-116,118,205,208,209,239,241,267] This was discussed briefly in Chapter 5 when Guild's theory of longitudinal flow of endolymph was considered.[93] It was shown that there is little or no scientific evidence to suggest that failure of the endolymph to drain through the saccus endolymphaticus is the cause of hydrops in man. Not only is there insufficient evidence for such an obstruction of flow, there is a good deal of opinion and some evidence to suggest that operative drainage of the sac does not achieve its purpose.[227] Schuknecht states, "I would expect endolymphatic surgery to *block* endolymph drainage — probably reversing the flow (if any) for the first few days, but it doesn't increase the vertigo during this period. Many cases with advanced hydrops have such severe membrane distortions that the outflow of endolymph can be blocked at the ductus reuniens, the saccule, the saccular duct, the utricular duct and the sinus of the endolyphatic duct. These are some of the reasons that sac surgery seems irrational to me. The sac operation and metabolic therapy have haunted us for over 50 years. It is doubtful whether they will endure. These are not logical therapies."*

Colman states, "Maybe the best that can be said for the saccus 'decompression' operation in which the area of dura is merely uncovered is that it is a placebo procedure with which useful comparisons can be made for those operations in which the endolymphatic sac is 'opened' or 'drained' or 'shunted.' For draining and shunting there is some rational basis albeit a

---

*H. Schuknecht, personal communication.

somewhat imaginative one, which lacks scientific and experimental confirmation. Perhaps one must ask again whether the consistent failure to control Meniere's disease by conservation operations designed to influence the endolymph 'hydrops' and 'increased pressure' are based on false assumptions."[48]
These critiques of endolymphatic sac surgery are further supported by most long-term results of the different operative techniques. As has been stressed before in all methods of treatment of Meniere's, the results have depended upon the length of follow-up. Glasscock states that most long-term follow-up series show only a 50 percent control of vertigo.[86] Alford put the figure at 66 percent but stated that in many of the reported series the follow-up has been too short or there has been a lack of controls, a poor experimental design to the investigations, and perhaps most significant of all, an illassorted group of patients upon which to operate.[5] The remarkable placebo effect of an operation has been investigated and described by Thomsen.[261]
It is perhaps not unfair to say that endolymphatic sac surgery has brought out all the difficulties inherent in diagnosing and managing Meniere's and in honestly assessing the results of treatment.

ESTABLISHED MENIERE'S — STAGE 4

The clinical picture in established Meniere's cases is one of incapacitating vertigo, often continuous tinnitus, and a loss of hearing in the affected ear at all frequencies. The audiogram is often flat, the loss may still be most pronounced in the low frequencies, or high tone involvement may have begun. Although fluctuation of hearing and tinnitus still occurs, they are now on a minor scale. Even at this stage the disease can be self-limiting, and no further progression may occur; however, this is unusual and not to be expected in an individual case.

The choice of treatment lies between active continuous drug therapy during all periods of relapse, linked with reduced dosage continuation therapy during remissions, and surgery. The aim of medical treatment is to suppress the vertigo and control the tinnitus; the condition is no longer reversible.

If vertiginous attacks continue, surgical treatment is indicated, and the operation of choice is selective vestibular nerve section. This procedure was first performed by the intracranial route by McKenzie in 1932[161] but has now been superseded by the middle cranial fossa approach.[85] This has given successful control of vertigo and preservation of hearing in the majority of cases. This is especially important in the unilateral case with severe uncontrolled vertigo without severe hearing loss. It is, however, a major operation requiring considerable skill and experience.[248]

Other methods of selective vestibular destruction using ultrasound or cryosurgery[8-10,117,289-291] are less reliable but have a definite place in those units which specialise in these techniques.

LATE MENIERE'S — STAGE 5

At the late Meniere's stage hearing in the affected ear is of no practical use to the patient, and tinnitus is often severe and continuous. As the hearing drops, so does the tendency to suffer from further vertigo attacks, but in some patients these attacks continue. When this is the case, medical treatment is often of very little help, and the patient may be almost totally incapacitated, partly from the actual results of the disease but also because of the severe somatopsychic effects. Repeated vertigo or the fear of repeated vertigo is not conducive to normal life.

The treatment of choice is surgical destruction of the labyrinth concerned. The operation was commenced and popularised by Cawthorne with his approach through the lateral semicircular canal.[42] The occasional failure of his technique to eradicate vestibular function led to the more radical techniques of transtympanic labyrinthectomy[153] and transcanal labyrinthectomy.[100,207] Pulec also advocated translabyrinthine section of the whole eighth nerve for intractable cases. Destruction of the labyrinth can also be achieved using ultrasound or cryosurgery, as previously stated.

While good medical management will usually control tinnitus, sometimes this is the major complaint and requires definite treatment. Barany described relief with intravenous procaine,[23] and Fowler used this in Meniere's with some success.[67] Intravenous lignocaine was suggested by Englesson[61] and used in Meniere's by Getrot.[77,78] This work was supported and continued by Melding[166] and by Shea and Harrell.[242] Melding and Goodey also suggested treatment with oral anticonvulsants. Their conclusion was that lignocaine was highly effective in suppressing tinnitus in patients with damage to, or degeneration of, the organ of Corti and less effective in other cases. In the group that benefitted from a trial dose of lignocaine, treatment with carbamazepine (Tegretol®) or diphenylhydantoin (Dilantin®) was likely to give good results.[167]

Surgical relief of tinnitus has also been advocated. Ferreri successfully treated a case by division of the cervical sympathetic chain,[63] and others have also reported improvement in, or abolition of, tinnitus following cervical sympathectomy.[88] Lempert advised excision of the tympanic plexus.[152]

BILATERAL MENIERE'S — STAGE 6

Perhaps the most difficult problems in the whole management of Meniere's arise when involvement of both inner ears is suspected or confirmed. This involvement can occur at any stage of the disorder but is extremely rare in the very early or early stages. Although Morrison states that 45 percent have bilateral involvement after twenty years,[180,181] this is not in keeping with personal experience or the experience of many workers in this field who put the figure nearer 10 percent.

The vast majority of clinicians agree that medical treatment should always precede surgical treatment, but there has been a tendency of late to operate much earlier upon cases that do not respond quickly and satisfactorily to medical measures. This is the result partly of the appreciation that the period of reversibility may be limited and partly upon the overenthusiastic short-term reports on the results of endolymphatic sac surgery. Indeed, surgery of this type has been recommended for bilateral Meniere's, although it is now accepted that it does little, if anything, to arrest the disease process particularly in the cochlea.

With evidence of bilateral disease, extreme caution should precede all advice advocating surgery. Labyrinthectomy on the severely deaf ear may occasionally be justifiable if the other ear only has very early and reversible hearing changes. Vestibular branch of eighth nerve section would be safer. Management must then, of course, be concentrated upon the control of the disease in the good ear.

If the patient has no useful hearing in one ear and is getting Meniere's attacks from the good ear, Pulec advocates the endolymphatic subarachnoid shunt operation.[209] Endolymphatic sac surgery for other stages of bilateral involvement has also been recommended and practised and has one great merit: it is unlikely to do any harm to the remaining auditory function in either ear. It is, in fact, extremely likely that the operation or operations act purely as a placebo effect. That such effects are common in Meniere's is supported by Thomsen and his co-workers.[260,261]

If there is bilateral involvement with more than minimal hearing loss in the better ear, the operation of choice is a bilateral cervical sympathectomy[1,102,103,278,283,285] This operation was suggested by Seymour and pioneered by Passe[194,195] and enjoyed considerable popularity for several years in papers by a number of workers.[1,53,89,90,102,156,276,278,285] It is very important in such cases to obtain any potential reversibility, of both cochlear and vestibular function, especially in the less affected ear. Consequently, operation, if decided upon, should not be delayed.

Although few long-term studies of sympathectomy have been published,[1,278] the results have been generally satisfactory with little evidence of sympathetic regeneration. It should be emphasized that many of these patients had reached the end of the road as far as treatment was concerned. Failure of sympathectomy to control the disease may be due to the following:

1. A functional reorganisation of the sympathetic pathways via intermediate sympathetic ganglia on the roots of the cervical plexus.[246] This reorganisation could be through preganglionic fibres left intact or by the phenomenon of collateral sprouting.[182]
2. The upper limit of the thoracicolumbar outflow may be as high as C7, so the usual stellatectomy will leave some of the pathway intact.

The patient with progressive bilateral Meniere's is indeed a challenge to any otological or neurootological team, but much can be done to help such unfortunate individuals by following the principles of treatment at the different stages that have already been outlined.

If, as the author believes and has indicated, Seymour's theory of the etiology is the one that best fits the clinical manifestations of Meniere's, as well as being most in harmony with the modern physiological findings, it seems appropriate that the application of this hypothesis presents no easy solution for the physician or surgeon treating this condition. It requires early referral of cases, early diagnosis, a considerable insight into the emotional and other problems present, a genuine ability to communicate fully with the patient (and other members of the team), and a personal commitment to each case for treatment to be satisfactory.

SUMMARY

Teamwork is essential for successful treatment of Meniere's and should be under the leadership of an interested (and dedicated) otologist or neurootologist. The approach to the problem in each case should be a holistic one, with the emphasis on general management. Practical psychiatric advice, as well as medical and surgical skills should be available to the team, backed up by skilled technical and nursing services, and with a definite commitment to a supportive as well as a treatment rôle.

Management depends largely upon what stage the disorder has reached when a definite diagnosis is first made. In stages 1 to 3 (very early, early, and intermediate), emphasis should be on obtaining total reversibility, or as great a degree of reversibility as is possible, as early as possible. Success in this respect should be relatively consistent in stages 1 and 2. In stage 3 there is some permanent impairment of both cochlear and vestibular function, and progression towards stage 4 (established Meniere's) is likely, with the optimum time for curative treatment fast running out. If operative treatment is to be considered, it should be on the basis of conservation of all remaining function. While many advocate endolymphatic sac surgery at this stage, it has no sound physiological basis, probably does not achieve the aim of ensuring endolymph drainage, and may well be little more than a placebo procedure.

Treatment of stage 4 consists of the control of vertigo by

prolonged drug therapy or by selective vestibular destruction using section of the vestibular nerve or ultrasonic or cryosurgical measures. Again, the emphasis is upon the conservation of all remaining auditory function.

In stage 5 (late Meniere's) the treatment of choice is surgical destruction of the affected labyrinth with no attempt to conserve any small degree of residual hearing. Tinnitus control of this stage (and stage 4 sometimes) is often necessary both before and after a destructive procedure.

Bilateral Meniere's (stage 6) poses special problems, and any surgery likely to increase hearing loss is strongly contraindicated. There may well be a place, at this stage, for bilateral cervical sympathectomy performed as early as possible.

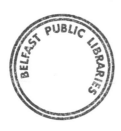

BIBLIOGRAPHY

1. Adams, D.A., and Wilmot, T.J. (1982). Ménière's disease: Long-term results of sympathectomy. *J Laryngol Otol, 96*:705-710.
2. Adour, K.K., Byl, F.M., Hilsinger, R.L., Jr., and Wilcox, R.D. (1980). Ménière's disease as a form of cranial polygánglionitis. *Laryngoscope, 90*:392-398.
3. Alfaro, V.R. (1958). Diagnostic significance of fullness in the ear. *JAMA, 166*:239-245.
4. Alford B.R. (1972). Ménière's disease: Criteria for diagnosis and evaluation of therapy for reporting. Report of the Sub-Committee on Equilibrium and its measurement. *Trans Am Acad Opthalmol Otolaryngol, 76*:1462-1464.
5. Alford, B.R., Cohn, A.M., and Igarashi, M. (1977). Current status of surgical decompression and drainage procedures upon the endolymphatic system. *Ann Otol Rhinol Laryngol, 86*:683-688.
6. Altmann, F., and Waltner, J.G. (1950). New investigations on the physiology of the labyrinthine fluids. *Laryngoscope, 60*:727-739.
7. Altmann, F., and Waltner, J.G. (1950). Further investigations on the physiology of the labyrinthine fluids. *Ann Otol Rhinol Laryngol, 59*:657-686.
8. Angell-James, J. (1965). Ultrasonic therapy for hydrops. *Laryngoscope, 75*:1552-1557.
9. Angell-James, J., Dalton, G.A., Bullen, M.A., Freundlich, H.F., and Hopkins, J.C. (1960). The ultrasonic treatment of Ménière's disease. *J Laryngol Otol, 74*:730-757.
10. Angell-James, J., Freundlich, H.F., Bullen, M.A., Wells, P.N.T., and Williams, D.P.C. (1964). The physical and biological properties of ultra-sound and clinical experience. *Acta Otolaryngol [Suppl], 192*: 134-138.

91

11. Antoli-Candela, F., Jr. (1976). The histopathology of Ménière's disease. *Acta Otolaryngol [Suppl.], 340.*
12. Arenberg, I.K. (1979). Endolymphatic sac valve implant surgery. *Laryngoscope [Suppl.] 17(7)*, Part 2: 1-53.
13. Arenberg, I.K., Marovitz, W.F., and Shambaugh, G.E., Jr. (1970). The role of the endolymphatic sac in the pathogenesis of endolymphatic hydrops in man. *Acta Otolaryngol [Suppl.] 275*:1-49.
14. Arenberg, I.K., Rask-Andersen, H., Wilbrand, H., and Stahle, J. (1977). The surgical anatomy of the endolymphatic sac. *Arch Otolaryngol, 103*:1-11.
15. Arnvig, J. (1947). Histological findings in case of Ménière's disease with remarks on pathologic-anatomical basis of this lesion. *Acta Otolaryngol, 35*:453-456.
16. Arroyo, J.A., and Hinchcliffe, R. (1977). Caloric test with oculogyral illusion as response. *J Laryngol Otol, 91*:309-321.
17. Arslan, M. (1953). Treatment of Ménière's syndrome by direct application of ultrasound waves to the vestibular system. *Proc. of 5th International Congress of Otolaryngology*, Amsterdam, pp.429-436.
18. Arslan, M. (1962). An improved technique of the ultrasonic irradiation of the vestibular apparatus by Ménière's disease. *Acta Otolaryngol, 55*:467-472.
19. Aschan, G., and Stahle, J. (1957). Nystagmus in Ménière's disease during attacks. *Acta Otolaryngol, 47*:189-201.
20. Ashcroft, M.T., Cruickshank, E.K., Hinchcliffe, R., Jones, W.I., Miall, W.E., and Wallace, J. (1967). A neurological ophthalmological and audiological survey of a suburban Jamaican community. *West Ind Med J, 16*:233-245.
21. Atkinson, M. (1962). Migraine and Ménière's disease. *Arch Otolaryngol, 75*:220-225.
22. Austin, D.F. (1981). Polytomography in Ménière's disease — an update. *Laryngoscope, 91*:1669-1675.
23. Barany, R. (1935). Die Beeinflussung des Ohrensausens durch intravenös injizierte Lokalanästhetica vorläufige Mitteilung. *Acta Otolaryngol, 23*:201-203.
24. Batsakis, J.G., and Nishiyama, R.H. (1962). Deafness with sporadic goiter. *Arch Otolaryngol, 76*:401-406.
25. Becker, G.D. (1979). Late syphilitic hearing loss: a diagnostic and therapeutic dilemma. *Laryngoscope, 89*:1273-1288.
26. Beentjes, B.I.J. (1972). The cochlear aqueduct and the pressure of cerebrospinal and endolabyrinthine fluids. *Acta Otolaryngol, 73*: 112-120.
27. Belal, A., Jr., and Linthicum, F.H., Jr. (1980). Pathology of congeni-

tal syphilitic labyrinthitis. *Am J Otololaryngol, 1*:109-118.

28. Berggren, S. (1949). Histological investigation of three cases with "Ménière" syndrome. *Acta Otolaryngol, 37*:30-36.

29. Black, R.J. (1982). Fluctuating hearing loss in W. African and W. Indian racial groups: Yaws, syphilis or Ménière's disease? (clinical records). *J Laryngol Otol, 96*:847-855.

30. Boettcher, A. (1869). Ueber den Aquaeductus vestibuli bei Katzen und Mervschen. *Arch Anat Physiol [Lpz], 372*-380.

31. Bosher, S.K. (1979). The nature of the negative endocochlear potentials produced by anoxia and ethacrynic acid in the rat and guinea-pig. *J Physiol, 293*:329-345.

32. Bosher, S.K. (1983). Personal communication.

33. Bosher, S.K., and Warren, R.L. (1971). A study of the electrochemistry and osmotic relationships of the cochlear fluids in the neonatal rat at the time of the development of the endocochlear potential. *J Physiol, 212*:739-761.

34. Bosher, S.K., and Warren, R.L. (1978). Very low calcium content of cochlear endolymph, an extra cellular fluid. *Nature, 273*:377-378.

35. Brackmann, D.E., and Anderson, R.G. (1980). Ménière's disease: Results of treatment with the endolymphatic subarachnoid shunt. *ORL, 42*:101-118.

36. Brain, W.R. (1963). Some unresolved problems of cervical spondylosis. *Br Med J, 1*:771-777.

37. Brown, M.R. (1949). The factor of heredity in labyrinthine deafness and paroxysmal vertigo (Ménière's syndrome). *Ann Otol Rhinol Laryngol, 58*:665-670.

38. Bull, J.W.D., Nixon, W.L.B., and Pratt, R.T.C. (1955). The radiological criteria and familial occurrence of primary basilar impression. *Brain, 78*:229-247.

39. Burian, K. (1952). Treatment by anaesthetic block in oto-rhino-laryngology. *Monatsschr Ohrenheilkd, 86*:109-112.

40. Busanny-Caspari, W., and Matzker, J. (1960). Neue Gesichtspunkte zur Histo-Pathologie des Morbus Meniere. *Z Laryngol Rhinol Otol, 39*:182-189.

41. Cawthorne, T. (1947). Ménière's disease *Ann Otol Rhinol Laryngol, 56*:18-38.

42. Cawthorne, T. (1956). Ménière's disease. *J Laryngol Otol, 70*:695-700.

43. Ceroni, T., and Franzoni, M. (1963). Aspetti psicosomatici della malattia di Ménière. *Ann Laringol [Torino], 62*:306-315.

44. Chou, J.T.Y. and Rodgers, K. (1962). Respiration of tissues lining the mammalian membranous labyrinth. *J Laryngol Otol, 76*:341-351.
45. Cinnamond, M.J. (1975). Eustachian tube function in Ménière's disease. *J Laryngol Otol, 89*:57-61.
46. Clemis, J.D., and Shambaugh, G.E. Jr. (1966). Preliminary experiences with operations on the endolymphatic sac. *Laryngoscope, 76*:1029-1041.
47. Coats, A.C. (1981). The summating potential and Ménière's disease. *Arch Otolaryngol, 107*:199-208.
48. Colman, B.H. (1982). Surgical treatment of Ménière's disease (editorial). *Clin Otolaryngology, 7*:363-365.
49. Craik, K.J.W. (1943). The nature of explanation. London.
50. Davis, H. (1957). Ménière's disease (editorial). *Br Med J, 2*:754-755.
51. Davis, H. (1957). Biophysics and physiology of the inner ear. *Physiol Rev, 37*:1-49.
52. De Kleyn, A., and Von Devivere, D. (1942). A new form of positional nystagmus. *Acta Otolaryngol, 30*:97-103.
53. Dix, M.R. (1956). Conservative surgery in the management of Ménière's disease. *J Laryngol Otol, 70*:686-694.
54. Dix, M.R. (1971). Disorders of balance: A recent clinical neuro-otological study. *Proc R Soc Med, 64 (2)*:857-860.
55. Dohlmann, G.F. (1976). On the mechanism of the Ménière attack. *Arch Otorhinolaryngol, 212*:301-307.
56. Dolowitz, D.A. (1979). Ménière's — an inner ear seizure. *Laryngoscope, 89*:67-77.
57. Edwards, C.H. (1973). In *Neurology of Ear, Nose and Throat Diseases*. London, Butterworths.
58. Eggermont, J.J., Don, M., and Brackmann, D.E. (1980). Electrocochleography and auditory brain stem electric responses in patients with pontine angle tumours. *Ann Otol Rhinol Laryngol [Suppl.], 75*:1-19.
59. Elies, W., and Plester, D. (1980). Basilar impression. *Arch Otolaryngol, 106*:232-233.
60. Enander, A., and Stahle, J. (1967). Hearing in Ménière's disease — a study of pure-tone audiograms in 334 patients. *Acta Otolaryngol, 64*:543-556.
61. Englesson, S., Larsson, B., Lindquist, N.G., Lyttkens, L., and Stahle, J. (1976). Accumulation of C-lidocaine in the inner ear. *Acta Otolaryngol, 82*:297-300.
62. Fernandez, C., and Hinojosa, R. (1974). Post natal development

of endo cochlear potential and stria vascularis in the cat. *Acta Otolaryngol, 78*:173-186.

63. Ferreri, G. (1903). La percezione acustica dopo gli interventi operative sull 'apparechio di transmissione del suono. *Arch Ital Otol, 14*:251-260.

64. Fick, I.A. van N. (1964). Decompression of the labyrinth. *Arch Otolaryngol, 79*:447-458.

65. Fick, I.A. van N. (1966). Ménière's disease: Aetiology and a new surgical approach: sacculotomy (decompression of the labyrinth). *J Laryngol Otol, 80*:288-306.

66. Fowler, E.P. Jr. (1949). Capillary circulation with changes in sympathetic activity; blood sludge from sympathetic stimulation. *Proc Soc Exp Biol Med, 72*:592-594.

67. Fowler, E.P. (1953). Intravenous procaine in the treatment of Ménière's disease. *Ann Otol Rhinol Laryngol, 62*:1186-1200.

68. Fowler, E.P. (1956). Intravascular agglutination of the blood: A factor in certain diseases and disorders of the ear. *Ann Otol Rhinol Laryngol, 65*:535-544.

69. Fowler, E.P., and Zeckel, A. (1952). Psychosomatic aspects of Ménière's disease. *JAMA, 148*:1265-1268.

70. Fowler, E.P., and Zeckel, A. (1953). Psychophysiological factors in Ménière's disease. *Psychosom Med, 15*:127-139.

71. Fraser, J.G., and Flood, L.M. (1982). An audiometric test for perilymph fistula. *J Laryngol Otol, 96*:513-519.

72. Fraysse, B.G., Alonso, A., and House, W.F. (1980). Ménière's disease and endolymphatic hydrops. Clinical histopathological correlations. *Ann Otol Rhinol Laryngol [Suppl.], 76*:1-22.

73. Frew, I.J.C., and Menon, G.N. (1976). Betahistine hydrochloride in Ménière's disease. *Postgrad Med J, 52*:501-503.

74. Fromm-Reichmann, F. (1937). Contributions to the psychogenesis of migraine. *Psychoanal Rev, 24*:26-33.

75. Furstenberg, A.C., Lashmet, F.H., and Lathrop, F. (1934). Ménière's symptom complex: Medical treatment. *Ann Otol Rhinol Laryngol, 43*:1035-1046.

76. Futaki, T., Kitahara, M., and Morimoto, M. (1977). A comparison of the furosimide and glycerol tests for Ménière's disease. *Acta Otolaryngol, 83*:272-278.

77. Gejrot, T. (1963). Intravenous Xylocaine in the treatment of attacks of Ménière's disease. *Acta Otolaryngol [Suppl.], 188*:190-195.

78. Gejrot, T. (1976). Intravenous Xylocaine in the treatment of attacks of

Ménière's disease. *Acta Otolaryngol, 82*:301-302.

79. Gellhorn, E. (1957). *Autonomic Imbalance and the Hypo-thalamus*. Minneapolis, U of Minnesota Press.

80. Gibson, W.P.R. (1979). In The physical and functional examination of the ear. In Scott-Browne: *Diseases of the Ear, Nose, and Throat*, 4th ed. vol. 2. London, Butterworths, pp.1-48.

81. Gibson, W.P.R., and Beagley, H.A. (1976). Trans-tympanic electrocochleography in the investigation of retro-cochlear disorders. *Rev Laryngol Otol Rhinol, 97 [Suppl.]*:507-516.

82. Gibson, W.P.R., Prasher, D.K., and Kilkenny, G.P.G. (1983). Diagnostic significance of trans-tympanic electrocochleography. *Ann Otol Rhinol Laryngol, 92*:155-159.

83. Gibson, W.P.R., Ramsden, R.T., Moffat, D.A. (1977). The immediate effects of naftidrofuryl on the human electrocochleogram in Ménière's disorder. *J Laryngol Otol, 91*:679-696.

84. Gill, N.W. (1968). On the treatment of vascular insufficiencies of the labyrinth with thymoxamine. *J Laryngol Otol, 82*:231-245.

85. Glasscock, M.E., and Miller, G.W. (1977). Middle fossa vestibular nerve section in the management of Ménière's disease. *Laryngoscope, 87*:529-541.

86. Glasscock, M.E., Miller, G.W., Drake, F.D., and Kanok, M.M. (1977). Surgical management of Ménière's disease with the endolymphatic subarachnoid shunt — a 5-year study. *Laryngoscope, 87*:1668-1675.

87. Golding-Wood, P.H. (1960). Water and salt balance in Ménière's disease. *J Laryngol Otol, 74*:480-488.

88. Golding-Wood, P.H. (1960). Ménière's disease and its pathological mechanism. *J Laryngol Otol, 74*:803-828.

89. Golding-Wood, P.H. (1960). Observations on sympathectomy in the treatment of Ménière's disease. *J Laryngol Otol, 74*:951-970.

90. Golding-Wood, P.H. (1969). The role of sympathectomy in the treatment of Ménière's disease. *J Laryngol Otol, 83*:741-770.

91. Gowers, W.R. (1893). *Diseases of the Nervous System*, 2nd ed., vol. 1. London, Churchill.

92. Groen, J. (1951). Emotional factors in the etiology of internal disease. The Isadore Friesner lecture. *J Mt. Sinai Hosp, 18*:71-89.

93. Guild, S.R. (1927). Circulation of endolymph. *Am J Anat, 39*:57-81.

94. Guilford, F.R. (1964). In The Treatment of Ménière's disease. In Fields, W.S., and Alford, B.R.: *Neurological Aspects of Auditory and Vestibular Disorders*. Springfield, Thomas.

95. Gussen, R. (1978). Melanocyte system of the endolymphatic duct and sac. *Ann Otol Rhinol Laryngol, 87*:175-179.

96. Gussen, R. (1982). Vascular mechanisms in Ménière's disease. *Arch Otolaryngol, 108*:544-549.

97. Hallpike, C.S., and Cairns, H. (1938). Observations on the pathology of Ménière's syndrome. *Proc Roy Soc Med, 31 (2)*:1317-1336.

98. Hallpike, C.S., and Cairns, H. (1938). Observations on the pathology of Ménière's syndrome. *J Laryngol Otol, 53*:625-655.

99. Hallpike, C.S., and Wright, A.J. (1940). On the histological changes in the temporal bones of a case of Ménière's disease. *J Laryngol Otol, 55*:59-66.

100. Hammerschlag, P.E., and Schuknecht, H.F. (1981). Transcanal labyrinthectomy for intractable vertigo. *Arch Otolaryngol, 107*:152-156.

101. Harker, L.A., and McCabe, B.F. (1980). In Paparella, M.M., and Shumrick, D.A.: *Otolaryngology*, 2nd ed. Philadelphia, Saunders, chap. 41, p. 1881.

102. Harrison, M.S. (1956). Conservative surgery in the management of Ménière's disease. *J Laryngol Otol, 70*:680-685.

103. Harrison, M.S., and Naftalin, L. (1968). In *Ménière's disease*. Springfield, Thomas.

104. Hegener, J. (1908). Klinische Beiträge zur Frage der akutem toxischen und infektiösen Neuritis des Nervus acusticus. *Z Ohrenheilkd, 55*:92-120.

105. Heron, J. (1983). Holistic medicine: A co-operative inquiry. *J R Soc Med, 76*:97-98.

106. Hicks, J.J., Hicks, J.N., and Cooley, H.N. (1967). Ménière's disease. *Arch Otolaryngol, 86*:610-613.

107. Hilger, J.A. (1950). Vasomotor labyrinthine ischemia. *Ann Otol Rhinol Laryngol, 59*:1102-1116.

108. Hinchcliffe, R. (1967). Headache and Ménière's disease. *Acta Otolaryngol, 63*:384-390.

109. Hinchcliffe, R. (1967). Personal and family medical history in Ménière's disease. *J Laryngol Otol, 81*:661-668.

110. Hinchcliffe, R. (1967). Emotion as a precipitating factor in Ménière's disease. *J Laryngol Otol, 81*:471-475.

111. Hommes, O.R., and Prick, J.J.G. (1968). Alopecia maligna. *Verh K Med Akad Wetensch*, 2nd Series, LVII-2, Amsterdam.

112. Hood, J.D., and Poole, J.P. (1966). Tolerance limit of loudness: Its clinical and physiological significance. *J Acoust Soc Am, 40*:47-53.

113. Hoogland, G.A. (1952). Treatment of Ménière's disease with cervical sympathetic block. *Acta Otolaryngol, 42*:379-386.

114. House, W.F. (1962). Subarachnoid shunt for drainage of endolym-

phatic hydrops: A preliminary report. *Laryngoscope, 72*:713-729.

115. House, W.F. (1964). Subarachnoid shunt for drainage of hydrops. *Arch Otolaryngol, 79*:338-354.

116. House, W.F. (1965). Subarachnoid shunt for drainage of hydrops. *Laryngoscope, 75*:1547-1551.

117. House, W.F. (1966). Cryosurgical treatment of Ménière's disease. *Arch Otolaryngol, 84*:616-629.

118. House, W.F., and Hitselberger, W.E. (1965). Endolymphatic subarachnoid shunt for Ménière's disease. *Arch Otolaryngol, 82*: 144-146.

119. Ireland, P.E., and Farkashidy, J. (1963). Electron microscopic studies of Ménière's disease: twelve fresh specimens taken at operation. *Trans Am Acad Opthalmol Otolaryngol, 67*:28-36.

120. Irvine, W.J., Luck, R.J., and Jacobey, J.A. (1965). Reversed blood flow in the vertebral arteries causing recurrent brain-stem ischaemia. *Lancet, 1*:994-996.

121. Janeke, C.E., Janeke, J.B., and Oosterveld, W.J. (1971). An improved version of the torsion-swing chair. *Ann Otol Rhinol Laryngol, 80*:229-232.

122. Johnson, L.F. (1954). Surgery of the sympathetic in Ménière's disease, tinnitus aurium and nerve deafness. *Arch Otolaryngol, 59*: 492-498.

123. Johnson, L.F., Whitelaw, G.P., and Strong, M.S., (1953). A review with comments on its treatment by sympathetic-nervous-system surgery. *Boston Med Q, 4*:1-6.

124. Jongkees, L.B.W. (1964). Medical treatment of Ménière's disease. *Acta Otolaryngol, [Suppl.], 192*:109-112.

125. Jongkees, L.B.W. (1980). Some remarks on Ménière's disease. *ORL, 42*:1-9.

126. Jongkees, L.B.W., Maas, J.P., and Philipszoon, A.J. (1962). Clinical nystagmography: A detailed study of electro-nystagmography in 341 patients with vertigo. *Pract Otorhinolaryngol (Basel), 24*:65-93.

127. Jongkees, L.B.W., and Philipszoon, A.J. (1964). The caloric test in Ménière's disease. *Acta Otolaryngol, [Suppl.], 192*:168-170.

128. Jorgensen, M.B. (1961). The inner ear in diabetes mellitus. *Arch Otolaryngol, 74*:373-381.

129. Jorgensen, M.B., and Buch, N.H. (1961). Studies on inner-ear function and cranial nerves in diabetes. *Acta Otolaryngol, 53*:350-364.

130. Joslin, E.P., Root, H.F., White, P., Marble, A., and Bailey, C.C. (1946). In *The Treatment of Diabetes Mellitus*, 8th ed. Philadelphia,

Lea & Febiger.

131. Kaldegg, A., Davys, M., and O'Neill, D. (1952). Migraine as a stress disorder. *Postgrad Med J, 28*:101-106.

132. Kane, R.J., O'Connell, A.F., and Morrison, A.W. (1982). Primary basilar impression: An aetiological factor in Ménière's disease. *J Laryngol Otol, 96*:931-936.

133. Kaseff, L.G., Perkins, R., and Hambley, W.H. (1981). Radiological techniques for small acoustic tumours — a re-evaluation. *Laryngoscope, 91*:63-70.

134. Kerr, A.G., and Smyth, G.D.L. (1976). Destruction of the endolymphatic sac in the cat. *J Laryngol Otol, 90*:841-843.

135. Kerr, A.G., Smyth, G.D.L., and Cinnamond, M.J. (1973). Congenital syphilitic deafness, *J Laryngol Otol, 87*:1-12.

136. Kerr, A.G., Smyth, G.D.L., and Landau, H.D. (1970). Congenital syphilitic labyrinthitis. *Arch Otolaryngol, 91*:474-478.

137. Kumura, R.S. (1976). Experimental pathogenesis of hydrops. *Arch Otorhino-laryngol, 212*:263-275.

138. Kitamura, K., Schuknecht, H.F., and Kimura, R.S. (1982). Cochlear hydrops in association with collapsed saccule and ductus reuniens. *Ann Otol Rhinol Laryngol, 91*:5-13.

139. Klockhoff, I. (1975). The effect of glycerin on fluctuant hearing loss. *Otolaryngol Clin N Am, 8*:345-355.

140. Klockhoff, I., and Lindblom, U. (1966). Endolymphatic hydrops revealed by glycerol test. *Acta Otolaryngol, 61*:459-462.

141. Klockhoff, I., Lindblom, U., and Stahle, J. (1974). Diuretic treatment of Ménière's disease. *Arch Otolaryngol, 100*:262-265.

142. Kobrak, F. (1920). Die Gejässerkrankungen des Ohrenlabyrinths und ihne Beziehungen zur Ménière schen Krankheit. *Berl Klin Wochenschr, 57*:185-188.

143. Kozarek, J.A., Sackett, J.F., and Arenberg, I.K. (1980). The value of multidirectional tomography in endolymphatic sac surgery. *Otolaryngol Clin N Am, 13*:665-670.

144. Larsen, H.C., Angelborg, C., and Hultcrantz, E. (1982). The effect of glycerol on cochlear blood flow. *ORL, 44*:101-107.

145. Larsen, H.C., Angelborg, C., and Hultcrantz, E. (1982). The effect of urea and mannitol on cochlear blood flow. *Acta Otolaryngol, 94*:249-252.

146. Lawrence, M. (1971). Blood flow through the basilar membrane capillaries. *Acta Otolaryngol, 71*:106-114.

147. Lawrence, M. (1971). The function of the spiral capillaries. *Laryn-*

goscope, 81:1314-1322.

148. Lawrence, M., and McCabe, B.F. (1959). Inner-ear mechanics and deafness: Special considerations of Ménière's syndrome. *JAMA, 171*:1927-1932.

149. Lawrence, M., Nuttall, A.L., and Burgio, P.A. (1977). Oxygen reserve and auto-regulation in the cochlea. *Acta Otolaryngol, 83*: 146-152.

150. Lawrence, M., Wolsk, D., and Litton, W.B. (1961). Circulation of the inner-ear fluids. *Ann Otol Rhinol Laryngol, 70*:753-776.

151. Lawrence, M., Wolsk, D., and McCabe, B.F. (1961). Fluid barriers within the otic capsule. *Trans Am Acad Ophthalmol Otolaryngol, 65*:246-254.

152. Lempert, J. (1946). Tympanosympathectomy. *Arch Otolaryngol, 43*:199-212.

153. Lempert, J. (1948). Lempert decompression operation for hydrops of the endolymphatic labyrinth in Ménière's disease. *Acta Otolaryngol, 47*:551-570.

154. Lermoyez, M. (1919). Le vertige qui fait entendre (angiospasme labyrinthique). *Presse Med, 27*:1-3.

155. Lermoyez, M. (1929). Le vertige qui fait entendre (angiospasme labyrinthique) *Ann Mal Oreille Larynx, 48*:575-583.

156. Lewis, R.S. (1956). Conservative surgery in the treatment of Ménière's disease. *J Laryngol Otol, 70*:673-679.

157. Lindsay, J.R. (1942). Labyrinthine dropsy and Ménière's disease. *Arch Otolaryngol, 35*:853-867.

158. Lindsay, J.R., Schuknecht, H.F., Neff, W.D., and Kimura, R.S. (1952). Obliteration of the endolymphatic sac and cochlear aqueduct. *Ann Otol Rhinol Laryngol, 61*:697-716.

159. Lindsay, J.R., and Schulthess, G. Von (1958). An unusual case of labyrinthine hydrops. *Acta Otolaryngol, 49*:315-324.

160. Lundquist, P.G., Kimura, R., and Wersall, J. (1963). Experiments in endolymph circulation. *Acta Otolaryngol, [Suppl.], 188*:198-201.

161. McKenzie, K. (1932). The intracranial section of the vestibular division of the eighth cranial nerve. *Trans Acad Med Toronto*, Nov. 15.

162. Marcussen, R.M., and Wolff, H.G. (1949). A formulation of the dynamics of the migraine attack. *Psychosom Med, 11*:251-256.

163. Martinez, D.M. (1972). The effect of Serc (betahistine hydrochloride) on the circulation of the inner ear in experimental animals. *Acta Otolaryngol, [Suppl.], 305*:29-47.

164. Mayer, O., and Fraser, J.S. (1936). Pathological changes in the ear in

late congenital syphilis. *J Laryngol Otol, 51*:755-778.

165. Means, J.H. (1948). *The Thyroid and its Diseases*, 2nd. ed., Philadelphia, Lippincott, pp.231-234.

166. Melding, P.S., Goodey, R.J., and Thorne, P.R. (1978). The use of intravenous lignocaine in the diagnosis and treatment of tinnitus. *J Laryngol Otol, 92*:115-121.

167. Melding, P.S., and Goodey R.J. (1979). The treatment of tinnitus with oral anticonvulsants. *J Laryngol Otol, 93*:111-122.

168. Ménière, E. (1880). Quelques considérations sur la maladie du Ménière. Paris, J.B. Baillière et Fils.

169. Ménière, P. (1861). Mémoire sur des lésions de l'oreille interne donnant lieu à des symptômes de congestion cérébrale apopliectiforme. *Gaz Méd de Paris*, 3 *16*:597-601.

170. Meyerhoff, W.L., Paparella, M.M., and Shea, D. (1978). Ménière's disease in children. *Laryngoscope, 88*:1504-1511.

171. Misrahy, G.A., de Jonge, B.R., Shinabarger, E.W., and Arnold, J.E. (1958). Effects of localised hypoxia on the electrophysiological activity of the cochlea of the guinea-pig. *J Acoust Soc Am, 30*:705-709.

172. Misrahy, G.A., Hildreth, K.M., Shinabarger, E.W., Clark, L.C., and Rice, E.A. (1958). Endolymphatic oxygen tension in the cochlea of the guinea-pig. *J Acoust Soc Am, 30*:247-250.

173. Misrahy, G.A., Hildreth, K.M., Shinabarger, E.W., and Gannon, W.J. (1958). Electrical properties of wall of endolymphatic space of the cochlea (guinea-pig). *Am J Physiol, 194*:396-402.

174. Misrahy, G.A., Shinabarger, E.W., and Arnold, J.E. (1958). Changes in cochlear endolymphatic oxygen availability, action potential and micro-phonics during and following asphyxia, hypoxia and exposure to loud sounds. *J Acoust Soc Am, 30*:701-704.

175. Mizukoshi, K., Ino, H., Ishikawa, K., Watanabe, Y., Yamazaki, H., Kato, I., Okubo, J., and Watanabe, I. (1979). Epidemiological survey of definite cases of Ménière's disease collected by the 17 members of the Ménière's Disease Research Committee of Japan in 1975-76. *Adv Otorhinolaryngol, 25*:106-111.

176. Moffat, D.A., Booth, J.R., and Morrison, A.W. (1979). Metabolic investigations in Ménière's disease. *J Laryngol Otol, 93*:545-561.

177. Moffat, D.A., Booth, J.R., and Morrison, A.W. (1981). Metabolic investigations in Ménière's disease. *J Laryngol Otol, 95*:905-913.

178. Montandon, A. (1954). A new technique for vestibular investigation. *Acta Otolaryngol, 44*:594-596.

179. Morgenstern, C., and Miyamoto, H. (1979). D.C. potential and K +

activity in experimental endolymphatic hydrops. *Arch Otorhinolaryngol, 222*:273-274.

180. Morrison, A.W. (1975). Management of sensorineural deafness. London and Boston, Butterworths, pp.145-174.
181. Morrison, A.W. (1981). Ménière's disease. *J R Soc Med, 74*:183-189.
182. Murray, J.G., and Thompson, J.W. (1956). Regeneration by collateral sprouting in the partially denervated superior cervical ganglion of the cat. *J Physiol, 131*:32p-33p.
183. Mygind, S.H., and Dederding, D. (1932). Significance of water metabolism in general pathology as demonstrated by experiments on ear. *Acta Otolaryngol, 17*:424-466.
184. Naftalin, L., and Harrison, M.S. (1958). Circulation of labyrinthine fluids. *J Laryngol Otol, 72*:118-136.
185. Naito, T. (1962). Clinical studies on Ménière's disease. *Rev Laryngol (Bordeaux), 83*:361-383.
186. Northfield, D.W.C. (1973). In *The Surgery of the Central Nervous System*. Oxford, Blackwell Scientific, pp.518-529.
187. Nylén, C.O. (1950). Positional nystagmus: A review and future prospects. *J Laryngol Otol, 64*:295-318.
188. Øigard, A., Thomsen, J., Jensen, J., and Dorph, S. (1975). The narrow vestibular aqueduct. An unspecified radiological sign? *Arch Otorhinolaryngol, 211*:1-4.
189. Oosterveld, W.J. (1970). The parallel swing. *Arch Otolaryngol, 91*:154-157.
190. Oosterveld, W.J. (1980). Ménière's disease, signs and symptoms. *J Laryngol Otol, 94*:885-894.
191. Opheim, O., and Flottorp, G. (1957). Ménière's disease: Some audiological and clinical observations. *Acta Otolaryngol, 47*:202-218.
192. Palva, T., Jauhiainen, T., Sjöblom, C.J., and Ylikoshi, J. (1978). Diagnosis and surgery of acoustic tumours. *Acta Otolaryngol, 86*:233-240.
193. Parving, A. (1976). Ménière's disease in childhood. *J Laryngol Otol, 90*:817-821.
194. Passe, E.R.G. (1951). Sympathectomy in relation to Ménière's disease, nerve deafness and tinnitus. *Proc Roy Soc Med, 44*:760-771.
195. Passe, E.R.G., and Seymour, J.C. (1948). Ménière's syndrome: Successful treatment by surgery on the sympathetic. *Br Med J, 2*:812-816.
196. Perlman, H.B., and Yamada, S. (1967). Autoregulation of the strial blood flow. 3rd symposium on the role of the vestibular organs in

space exploration. N.A.S.A. SP-152.

197. Permin, P.M., and Poulsen, H. (1957). Ménière's disease: Follow-up on 371 patients treated in hospital by conservative measures. *Acta Otolaryngol, 47*:219-230.

198. Pietrantoni, L., and Iurato, S. (1960). Some initial electron microscope investigation of a case of Ménière's syndrome. *Acta Otolaryngol, 52*:15-26.

199. Pilsbury, H.C., and Shea, J.J. (1979). Luetic hydrops: Diagnosis and treatment. *Laryngoscope, 89*:1135-1144.

200. Plantenga, K.F., and Browning, G.G. (1979). The vestibular aqueduct and endolymphatic sac and duct in endolymphatic hydrops. *Arch Otolaryngol, 105*:546-552.

201. Pollard, T.J., Smith, C.A., and Brummett, R. (1981). The effects of low dose ethacrynic acid on the guinea-pig cochlea with special reference to normal variations in the stria vascularis. *Acta Otolaryngol, 92*:249-258.

202. Portmann, G. (1927). Surgical treatment by opening the saccus endolymphaticus. *Arch Otolaryngol, 6*:309-315.

203. Portmann, M., Le Bert, G., and Aran, J.M. (1967). Potentiels cochléaires obtenus chez l'homme en dehors de toute intervention chirugicale. *Rev Larngol (Bordeaux), 88*:157-164.

204. Poulsen, H. (1966). Thyrotrophic and thyroid hormone control of the inner ear with special reference to myxoedema and Ménière's disease. In Ashboe-Hansen: *Hormones and Connective Tissue.* Copenhagen, Munksgaard.

205. Pulec, J.L. (1969). The surgical treatment of vertigo. *Laryngoscope, 79*:1783-1822.

206. Pulec, J.L. (1972). Ménière's disease: Results of a two and one-half year study of etiology, natural history and results of treatment. *Laryngoscope, 82*:1703-1715.

207. Pulec, J.L. (1974). Labyrinthectomy: Indications, technique and results. *Laryngoscope, 84*:1552-1571.

208. Pulec, J.L. (1977). Indications for surgery in Ménière's disease. *Laryngoscope, 87*:542-556.

209. Pulec, J.L. (1981). Endolymphatic subarachnoid shunt for Ménière's disease in the only hearing ear. *Laryngoscope, 91*:771-783.

210. Quaranta, A., Amoroso, C., Ettorre, G.C., and Violante, F. (1982). Clinical and radiological findings in subjects with unilateral Ménière's disorder. *Clin Otolaryngology, 7*:29-34.

211. Rauch, S. (1966). Membrane problems of the inner ear and their sig-

nificance. *J Laryngol Otol, 80*:1144-1155.

212. Rinkel, H.J., Randolph, T.G., and Zeller, M. (1950). In *Food Allergy*. Springfield, Thomas.

213. Rollin, H. (1940) Zur Kenntnis des labyrinth-hydrops und des durch ihn bedingten Ménière. *Hals-Nasen-Ohrenarzt (Teil 1), 31*:73-109.

214. Rosen, S. (1951). Surgery in Ménière's disease: A new operation which preserves the labyrinth: report of cases. *Ann Otol Rhinol Laryngol, 60*:657-667.

215. Ryan, G.M.S., and Cope, S. (1955). Cervical vertigo, *Lancet, 2*:1355-1358.

216. Sadé, J. (1981). Ménière's disease. *J Laryngol Otol, 95*:261-271.

217. Schayer, R.W. (1959). Catabolism of physiological quantities of histamine *in vivo*. *Physiol Rev, 39*:116-126.

218. Schayer, R.W. (1961). Significance of induced histamine in physiology and pathology. *Chemotherapia, 3*:128-136.

219. Schayer, R.W. (1962). Evidence that induced histamine is an intrinsic regulator of the microcirculatory system. *Am J Physiol, 202*: 66-72.

220. Schayer, R.W. (1963). Induced synthesis of histamine, microcirculation regulation and the mechanism of action of the adrenal glucocorticoid hormones. *Prog Allergy, 7*:187-212.

221. Schilder, P. (1933). The vestibular apparatus in neurosis and psychosis. *J Nerv Ment Dis, 78*:1-23, 137-164.

222. Schindler, R.A. (1979). The ultra-structure of the endolymphatic sac in Ménière's disease. *Adv Otorhinolaryngol, 25*:127-133.

223. Schmidt, P.H., Brunsting, R.L., and Antvelink, J.B. (1979). Ménière's disease: Etiology and natural history. *Acta Otolaryngol, 87*:410-412.

224. Schuknecht, H.F. (1963). Ménière's disease: A correlation of symptomatology and pathology. *Laryngoscope, 73*:651-665.

225. Schuknecht, H.F. (1969). Cupulolithiasis. *Arch Otolaryngol, 90*: 765-778.

226. Schuknecht, H.F. (1976). Pathophysiology of endolymphatic hydrops. *Arch Otorhinolaryngol, 212*:253-262.

227. Schuknecht, H. (1977). Pathology of Ménière's disease as it relates to the sac and tack procedures. *Ann Otol Rhinol Laryngol, 86*:677-682.

228. Schuknecht, H.F., Benitez, J.T., and Beekhuis, J. (1962). Further observations on the pathology of Ménière's disease. *Ann Otol Rhinol Laryngol, 71*:1039-1053.

229. Schuknecht, H.F., and Seifi, A. El. (1963). Experimental observations on the fluid physiology of the inner ear. *Ann Otol Rhinol Laryngol, 72*:687-712.

230. Sellick, P.M., and Johnstone, B.M. (1972). The electrophysiology of the saccule. *Pflüigers Arch, 336*:28-34.

231. Sellick, P.M., Johnstone, J.R., and Johnstone, B.M. (1972). The electrophysiology of the utricle. *Pflüigers Arch, 336*:21-27.

232. Selters, W.A., and Brackmann, D.E. (1977). Acoustic tumour detection with brain stem electric response audiometry. *Arch Otolaryngol, 103*:181-187.

233. Seymour, J.C. (1954). Observations on the circulation in the cochlea. *J Laryngol Otol, 68*:689-711.

234. Seymour, J.C. (1960). The aetiology, pathology and conservative surgical treatment of Ménière's disease. *J Laryngol Otol, 74*:599-627.

235. Seymour, J.C., and Tappin, J.W. (1951). The effect of sympathetic stimulation upon the cochlear microphonic potentials. *Proc R Soc Med, 44*:755-759.

236. Seymour, J.C., and Tappin, J.W. (1953). Some aspects of the sympathetic nervous system in relation to the inner ear. *Acta Otolaryngol, 43*:618-635.

237. Shambaugh, G.E. (1909). Uber Bau und Funktion des Epithels un Sulcus spiralis externus. *Z Ohrenheilk, 58*:280-287.

238. Shambaugh, G.E. Jr. (1940). Diplacusis: A localising symptom of disease of the organ of Corti. *Arch Otolaryngol, 31*:160-184.

239. Shambaugh, G.E. Jr. (1966). Surgery of the endolymphatic sac. *Arch Otolaryngol, 83*:305-315.

240. Shapiro, S.L. (1936). Vertigo as syndrome in vascular disease. *Illinois Med J, 70*:512-515.

241. Shea, J.J. (1966). Teflon film drainage of the endolymphatic sac. *Arch Otolaryngol, 83*:316-319.

242. Shea, J.J., and Harell, M. (1978). Management of tinnitus aurium with lidocaine and carbamazepine. *Laryngoscope, 88*:1477-1484.

243. Siirala, V., Siltala, P., and Lumio, J.S. (1965). Psychological aspects of Ménière's disease. *Acta Otolaryngol, 59*:350-357.

244. Sjöberg, A. (1963). Treatment of Ménière's disease by ultrasonic irradiation. (physical, experimental and clinical studies). *Acta Otolaryngol [Suppl.], 178*.

245. Sjöberg, A. (1964). Clinical experience from the treatment of Ménière's disease. *Acta Otolaryngol [Suppl.], 192*:139-153.

246. Skoog, T. (1947). Ganglia in the communicating rami of the cervical

sympathetic trunk. *Lancet, 2*:457-460.
247. Smyth, G.D.L., Kerr, A.G., and Cinnamond, M.J. (1976). Deafness due to syphilis. *J Otolaryngol Soc Aust, 4*:36-40.
248. Smyth, G.D.L., Kerr, A.G., and Gordon, D.S. (1976). Vestibular nerve section for Ménière's disease. *J Laryngol Otol, 90*:823-831.
249. Snyder, J.M. (1982). Predictability of the glycerin test in the diagnosis of Ménière's disease. *Clin Otolaryngol, 7*:389-397.
250. Sørensen, H. (1959). Ménière's syndrome in a seven year old girl. *J Laryngol Otol, 73*:346-350.
251. Sørensen, H., and Andersen, M.S. (1976). The effect of ultrasound in Ménière's disease. *Acta Otolaryngol, 82*:312-315.
252. Sørensen, H., and Andersen, M.S. (1979). Long term results of ultrasonic irradiation in Ménière's disease. *Clinical Otolaryngology, 4*:125-129.
253. Spencer, J.T. (1973). Hyperlipoproteinemias in the etiology of inner ear disease. *Laryngoscope, 83*:639-678.
254. Spencer, J.T. (1975). Hyperlipoproteinemia and inner ear disease. *Otolaryngol Clin N Am, 8*:483-492.
255. Stahle, J., and Wilbrand, H. (1974). The vestibular aqueduct in patients with Ménière's disease. *Acta Otolaryngol, 78*:36-48.
256. Stephens, S.D.G. (1975). Personality tests in Ménière's disorder. *J Laryngol Otol, 89*:479-490.
257. Sterkers, O., Saumon, G., Toan-ba-huy, P., and Amiel, C. (1982). K Cl and H$_2$O entry in endolymph, perilymph and cerebro spinal fluid in the rat. *Am J Physiol, 243* (Renal fluid electrolyte Physiol 12) F, 173-180.
258. Taylor, I.G., and Irwin, J. (1978). Some audiological aspects of diabetes mellitus. *J Laryngol Otol, 92*:99-113.
259. Thomsen, J., Bech, P., Geisler, A., Prytz, S., Rafaelsen, O.J., Vendsborg, P., and Kilstorff, K. (1976). Lithium treatment of Ménière's disease. *Acta Otolaryngol, 82*:294-296.
260. Thomsen, J, Bech, P., Prytz, S., Vendsborg, P., and Zilstorff, K. (1979). Ménière's disease: Lithium treatment (demonstration of placebo effect in a double blind cross-over trial). *Clin Otolaryngol, 4*:119-123.
261. Thomsen, J., Bretlau, P., Tos, M., Johnsen, N.J. (1981). Placebo effect in surgery for Ménière's disease. *Acta Otolaryngol, 107*:271-277.
262. Thomsen, J., and Vesterhauge, S. (1979). A critical evaluation of the glycerol test in Ménière's disease. *J Otolaryngol, 8*:145-150.
263. Tjernstrom, O. (1974). Middle ear mechanics and alternobaric ver-

tigo. *Acta Otolaryngol, 78*:376-384.

264. Tjernström, O. (1977). Effects of middle ear pressure on the inner ear. *Acta Otolaryngol, 83*:11-15.

265. Torok, N. (1977). Old and new in Ménière's disease. *Laryngoscope, 87*:1870-1877.

266. Tumarkin, A. (1966). Thoughts on the treatment of labyrinthopathy. *J Laryngol Otol, 80*:1041-1053.

267. Turner, J.S., Saunders, A.Z., and Per-Lee, J.H. (1973): A 10-year profile of Ménière's disease and endolymphatic shunt surgery. *Laryngoscope, 83*:1816-1824.

268. Vernet, M. (1920). Le vertige et son traîtement par l'adrénaline. *Presse Med, 28*:462-464.

269. Watanabe, . (1981). Ménière's disease in males and females. *Acta Otolaryngol, 91*:511-514.

270. Weille, F.L. (1967). Microcirculation and fluid physiology of the inner ear correlated with Ménière's disease. *Laryngoscope, 77*: 2063-2076.

271. Weille, F.L. (1968). Hypoglycaemia in Ménière's disease. *Acta Otolaryngol, 87*:555-557.

272. Wiet, R.J., Kazan, R., and Shambaugh, G.E. (1981). An holistic approach to Ménière's disease. Medical and surgical management. *Laryngoscope, 91*:1647-1662.

273. Williams, H.L. (1952). *Ménière's Disease*. Springfield, Thomas.

274. Williams, H.L. Jr. (1965). A review of the literature as to the physiologic dysfunction of Ménière's disease: A new hypothesis as to its fundamental cause. *Laryngoscope, 75*:1661-1689.

275. Wilmot, T.J. (1957). Labyrinthine vascular disorders. *Ulster Med J, 26*:41-50.

276. Wilmot, T.J. (1961). Sympathectomy for inner-ear vascular insufficiency. *J Laryngol Otol, 75*:259-267.

277. Wilmot, T.J. (1966). The application of modern vestibulometry to the problem of vertigo. *J Laryngol Otol, 80*:1156-1172.

278. Wilmot, T.J. (1969). Sympathectomy for Ménière's disease — a long term review. *J Laryngol Otol, 83*:323-331.

279. Wilmot, T.J. (1970). A method of vestibular analysis. *J Laryngol Otol, 84*:1033-1047.

280. Wilmot, T.J. (1971). An objective study of the effect of betahistine hydrochloride on hearing and vestibular function tests in patients with Ménière's disease. *J Laryngol Otol, 85*:369-373.

281. Wilmot, T.J. (1972). The effect of betahistine hydrochloride in

Ménière's disease. *Acta Otolaryngol [Suppl], 305*:18-21.
282. Wilmot, T.J. (1973). Vestibular analysis in vestibular neuronitis. *J Laryngol Otol, 87*:239-251.
283. Wilmot, T.J. (1974). Otological balance. *Proc R Soc Med, 67*:331-336.
284. Wilmot, T.J. (1974). Vestibular analysis in Ménière's disease. *J Laryngol Otol, 88*:295-306.
285. Wilmot, T.J. (1979). Review: Ménière's disorder. *Clin Otolaryngol, 4*:131-143.
286. Wilmot, T.J., and Menon, G.N. (1976). Betahistine in Ménière's disease. *J Laryngol Otol, 90*:833-840.
287. Wilmot, T.J., and Seymour, J.C. (1960). Diagnosis and treatment of vascular insufficiency causing perceptive deafness. *Lancet, 1*: 1098-1102.
288. Wolff, H.H. (1963). The significance of psychosomatic symptoms as seen in psychotherapy. *Acta Psychother, 11*:323-332.
289. Wolfson, R.J. (1963). The treatment of various forms of vertigo by ultrasonic radiation. *Laryngoscope, 73*:673-682.
290. Wolfson, R.J., Cutt, R.A., Ishiyama, E. (1966). Cryosurgery of the labyrinth — preliminary report of a new surgical procedure. *Laryngoscope, 76*:733-757.
291. Wolfson, R.J., and Ishiyama, E. (1974). Current status of labyrinthine cryosurgery. *Laryngoscope, 84*:757-765.
292. Wright, A.J. (1937). Aural vertigo: A clinical study. *Proc R Soc Med, 31*:87-91.
293. Wright, A.J. (1938). Labyrinthine giddiness: Its nature and treatment. *Br Med J, 1*:668-670.
294. Wright, A.J. (1946). President's address (cochlear deafness). *Proc R Soc Med, 39*:265-267.
295. Yamashita, T., and Schuknecht, H.F. (1982). Apical endolymphatic hydrops. *Arch Otolaryngol, 108*:463-466.
296. Zechner, G., and Altmann, F. (1969). Histological studies on the human endolymphatic duct and sac. *Prac Otorhinolaryngol (Basel), 31*:65-83.

INDEX